Shoulder Arthroscopy

Shoulder Arthroscopy

Timothy D Bunker

BSc. MB BS(Hons), MCh (Orth), FRCS, FRCSEd

Consultant Orthopaedic Surgeon,
Princess Elizabeth Orthopaedic Hospital, Exeter,
and the Royal Devon and Exeter Hospital, Exeter, Devon, UK

W Angus Wallace

MB ChB, FRCSEd, FRCSEd Orth,

Professor of Orthopaedic and Accident Surgery,
University of Nottingham,
Nottingham, UK

MARTIN DUNITZ

First published in the United Kingdom in 1991
by Martin Dunitz Ltd, 7–9 Pratt Street, London NW1 0AE

British Library Cataloguing in Publication Data
Bunker, Timothy D.
Shoulder arthroscopy.
1. Man. Joints. Arthroscopic surgery 2. Man. Joints. Diagnosis. Arthroscopy
I. Title II. Wallace, W. A.
617.472059

ISBN 0-94826-963-4

Typeset by Scribe Design, Gillingham, Kent
Printed and bound in Singapore by Times Offset Pte. Ltd

Contents

Acknowledgments vii

Introduction 1

1 Extracapsular anatomy for shoulder arthroscopy 9

2 Assessment of the shoulder 25

3 Imaging the shoulder 41
Steven Austin, MB BS, FRCR

4 Clinical procedure 51

5 Normal arthroscopic examination 75

6 Abnormal findings 99

7 Arthroscopic surgery 123

8 Arthroscopic subacromial decompression 131

9 Arthroscopic management of traumatic shoulder dislocation 141

References 157

Further reading 161

Index 163

Acknowledgments

I would like to acknowledge the encouragement that has been given to me over the last ten years in developing my interest in shoulder arthroscopy: in particular the original help from Gordon Bannister, Harry Griffiths and Christopher Ackroyd in Bristol, further encouragement and my first arthroscopic camera from Professor Robin Ling in Exeter, guidance in the practicalities of shoulder arthroscopy from Professor Angus Wallace in Nottingham and Ian Bayley in London. Finally I would like to acknowledge the help I have had from the Porritt Fellowship of the Royal College of Surgeons of England which enabled me to make two visits to the United States, and from the following surgeons who gave me the benefit of their time and their wisdom: Dr Wiley and Dr Ogilvie Harris (Toronto), Dr Hawkins (London), Dr Matthews (Baltimore), Dr Rose (New York), Dr Johnson, Dr Schneider and Dr Detrisac (Lansing, Michigan), Dr Curtis (San Antonio, Texas) and Clive Warren-Smith (RAF Wroughton).

TDB

I have been delighted to assist in editing this book which has been written mainly by Tim Bunker. We have over the last five years learnt from each other, and the Nottingham Orthopaedic Residents have been amused by our arthroscopic efforts. I am particularly grateful to Dr Murray Wiley and Dr Bob Jackson in Toronto and to Ian Bayley in London who have helped me start my shoulder arthroscopic practice. Above all, however, I am grateful to the Operating Department theatre staff who have so patiently assisted us with our efforts, and also to the Orthopaedic Residents who have held the arms in the past before we started to use a 'Shoulder Holder'.

WAW

Sources

The authors wish to acknowledge the following for their kind permission to reproduce material:
Instrument Makar (Figures 4.3, 4.4); Schutt (Figure 4.5); Zimmer (Figure 4.8); the Editors of *The Journal of Bone and Joint Surgery* (Figures 5.19, 9.4); MA Hutson, *Sports Injury: Recognition and Management,* Oxford University Press (Figures 2.1, 2.2, 2.10–2.12, 2.13, 2.14).

Introduction

The decade of the 1980s has seen a spectacular growth in the area of shoulder arthroscopy and there is no doubt that this trend will continue into the next decade. The reason for this parallels the growth of knee arthroscopy during the late 1960s, the decade of the 1970s and the early part of the 1980s. The initial reason that shoulder arthroscopy took off was that it revolutionized the diagnosis of shoulder disorders, previously a realm that could only be mastered by the elite few who had made shoulder surgery their superspecialty. One such expert was Cyriax who encapsulated the attitude of most physicians thus: 'Many doctors regard disorders of the shoulder as uninteresting, undiagnosable, and incurable, but tending to recover in the end. Nothing could be further from the truth.' The arthroscope gives the surgeon an extremely powerful tool which not only assists in diagnosis, but by a process of feedback hones the surgeon's own clinical diagnostic acumen, giving an ability to diagnose shoulder disorders more accurately than the superspecialists ever could from outside the joint.

This book aims to open up this inner world of the shoulder joint and to stimulate interest in conditions around the shoulder. The book is aimed both at surgeons in training and also those experienced surgeons who are either shoulder surgeons who would like to be able to arthroscope the shoulder, or experienced arthroscopists who would like to develop a special interest in the shoulder.

Indications

Initially shoulder arthroscopy was used for diagnostic purposes alone. Such studies soon showed that clinical diagnosis was often incorrect and that shoulder arthroscopy could diagnose many conditions accurately. Cofield[1] reviewed 74 diagnostic arthroscopies and found that in 32 per cent, arthroscopy was important in making, confirming or modifying the diagnosis or in altering the course of treatment. In a further 45 per cent, it was optional and in only 23 per cent was it unnecessary. In trying to establish which modality gave a firm diagnosis, Cofield found that arthroscopy was twice as accurate as a combination of history, examination and routine radiographs.

The author's experience with the first 50 shoulder arthroscopies[2] was similar. In 27 cases out of 50, the diagnosis was changed or refined. In particular, dual or even triple pathology was found, and unexpected rotator cuff tears and loose bodies were not uncommon findings. Such a high diagnostic score has brought some shoulder surgeons to contemplate the need for shoulder arthroscopy in the majority of patients presenting with significant shoulder disorders. Logistically of course, this is not possible and so we have to consider which particular groups of patient can benefit most by diagnostic shoulder arthroscopy. There are four groups in whom shoulder arthroscopy is most helpful:

- *Patients aged 18–35, with recurrent shoulder discomfort following trauma*: It is becoming clearer that pain following trauma to the shoulder in young people is often due to instability. Rowe and Zarins' classic paper[3] describing transient subluxation and the dead arm syndrome initially brought this to the attention of the general orthopaedist, but this can be a difficult diagnosis to confirm.

Shoulder arthroscopy can be useful in this group, particularly if a Bankart lesion is present.

Damage to the inferior glenohumeral ligament, with or without a Bankart lesion, and damage to the middle glenohumeral ligaments are further pointers. There may be a Hill–Sachs lesion on the humeral head, some of which may be cartilaginous only, and therefore not show up on a Stryker Notch (West Point) radiograph. A loose body in the joint is most commonly associated with a Hill–Sachs lesion following an episode of dislocation, and damage to the anterior glenoid rim may be a further indication of recurrent subluxation.

Just as important as shoulder arthroscopy in this group is the examination under anaesthetic (EUA). This is a load and shift test and is described on page 36. To many surgeons, the EUA is actually more important than arthroscopy in recurrent subluxation. Certainly it should never be omitted. EUA should be performed before the arthroscopy, as it is easier in a fresh joint, before distension has been carried out. The problem with performing the EUA first is that it may cause intra-articular bleeding, but this can be controlled by adequate lavage (Figure A).

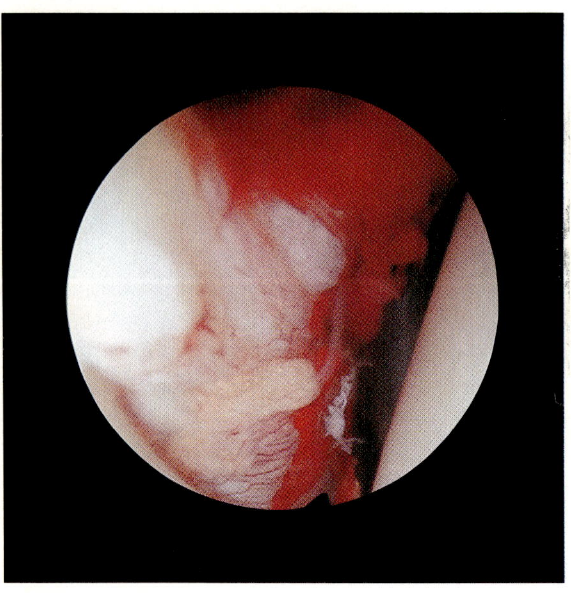

Figure A

Bleeding from a Bankart lesion following examination under anaesthetic can be controlled by lavage.

■ *Patients over 35, with chronic subacromial impingement*: To the shoulder surgeon, the painful arc is one of the most common presentations. Typically, patients complain of a painful arc of movement in the range of 70 to 120 degrees of elevation. If this does not settle within six months, with either physiotherapy or local installation of one injection of steroid, then arthroscopy is indicated (Chapter 8).

In particular, the surgeon will be looking for evidence of a rotator cuff tear (Figures B and C). Arthroscopically, the insertion of both supraspinatus (Figure D) and infraspinatus can be seen at the synovial reflection onto the humeral neck. Supraspinatus inserts onto the greater tuberosity behind the tunnel of the long head of biceps, the tendon being used as a landmark. Infraspinatus inserts onto the bare area of the posterior humeral head (Figure E).

The arthroscopist has the advantage over the radiologist in that the superior surface of the rotator cuff can be visualized as well, by performing a bursal endoscopy. The classic impingement lesion, an area of 'hairy degeneration' of the superior surface of the rotator cuff, may be seen (Figure F), or there may be a partial tear or ruffling up of the cuff. Any abnormality of the cuff can be probed, giving further tactile information. Partial thickness tears, which would not be visualized arthrographically, or areas of inflammation can be seen (Figure G) and probed. Tendinitis of the long head of biceps (Figure H) may be a marker of impingement and cuff tear.

■ *Atypical shoulder pain*: In the past, this had to be managed empirically, for a definite diagnosis could not be made. Under these

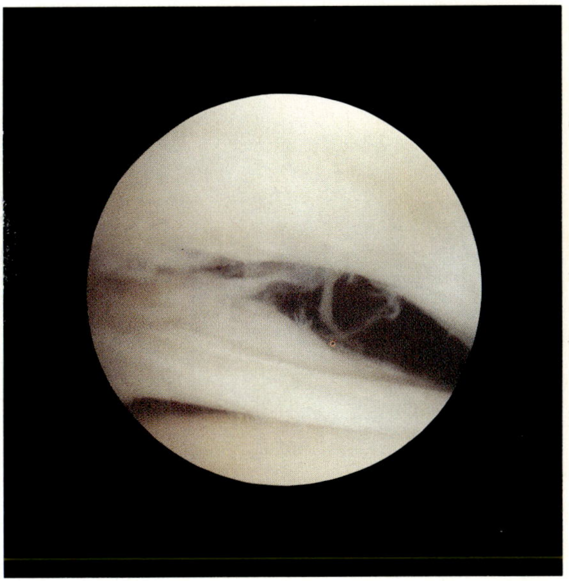

Figure B

A full thickness rotator cuff tear above the humeral head.

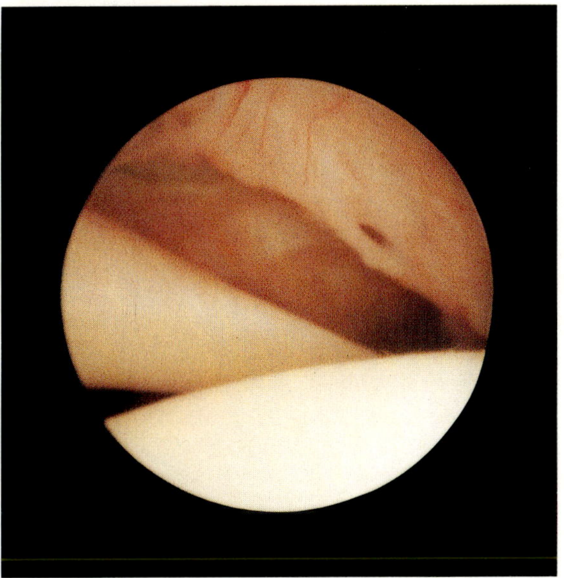

Figure C

The rolled mature edge of a rotator cuff tear next to the long head of the biceps tendon.

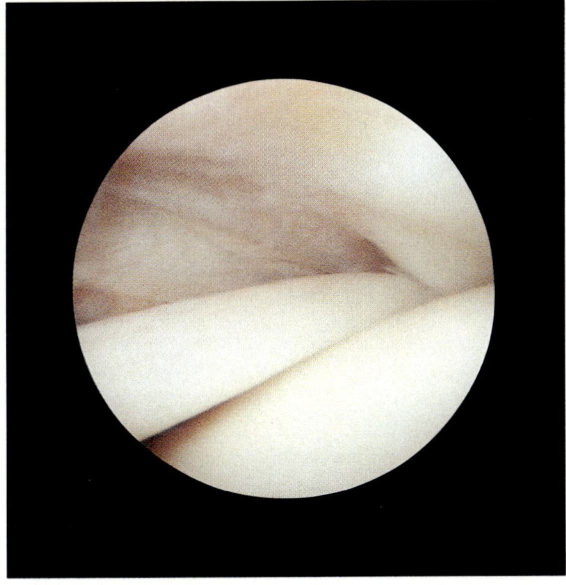

Figure D

The insertion of supraspinatus next to the long head of biceps.

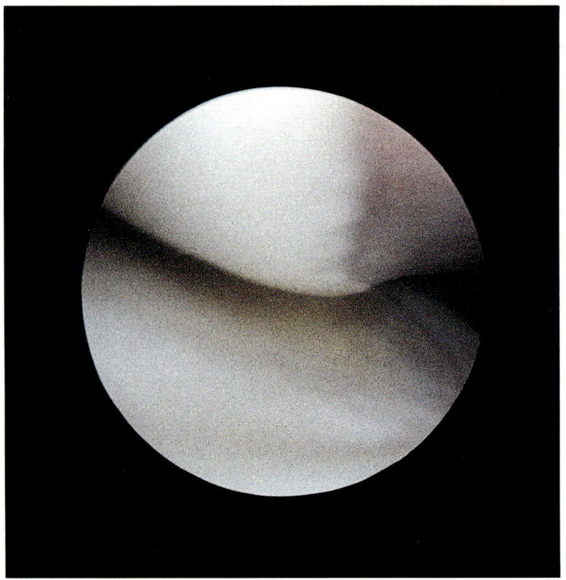

Figure E

The bare area of the humeral head.

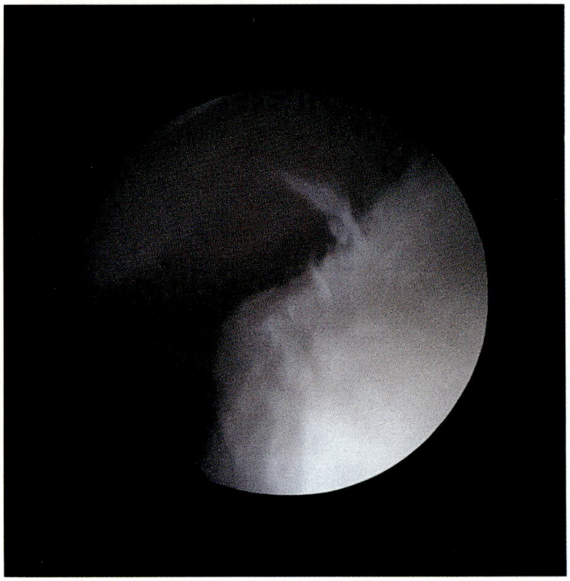

Figure F

The impingement lesion, a 'hairy degeneration' of the superior surface of the rotator cuff.

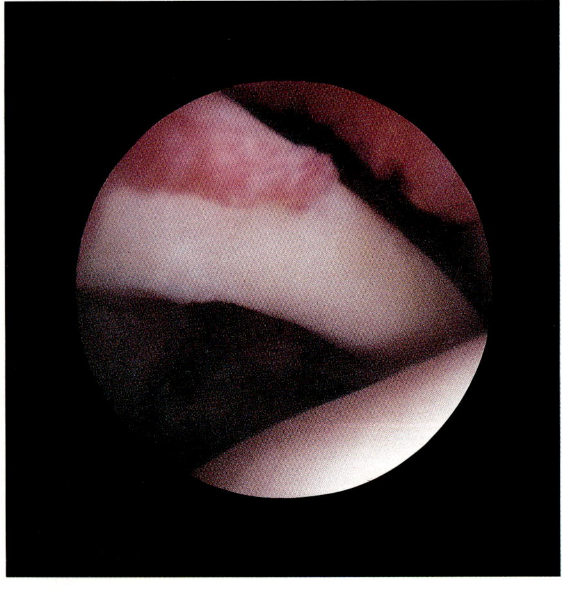

Figure G

Inflammation of a partial thickness rotator cuff tear seen above an equally inflamed biceps tendon.

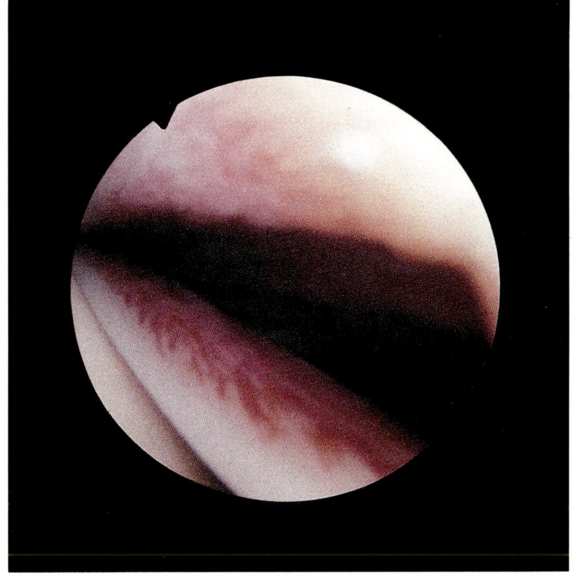

Figure H

Synovitis of the superior half of the biceps tendon.

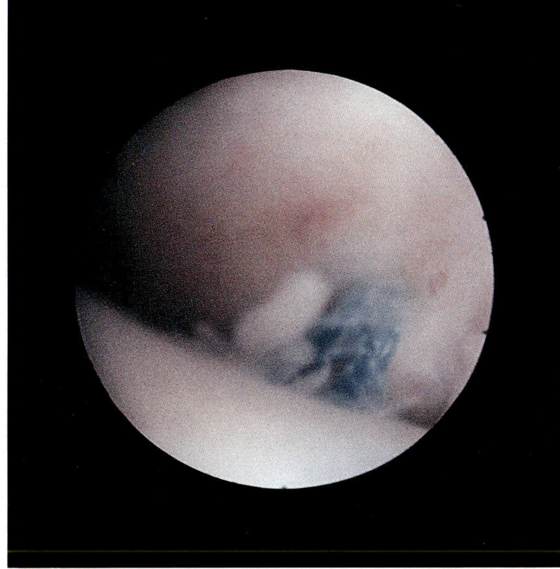

Figure I

Repairs of the rotator cuff can be difficult to see (and therefore to photograph). Seen here is an Ethibond suture of a rotator cuff repair just above the long head of the biceps tendon.

circumstances, arthroscopy can be of great value. In particular, the following diagnoses can often be missed clinically:

— glenoid labral tears, which may give intermittent shoulder pain or unpredictable locking or catching of the joint
— instability with no good history of initial dislocation
— loose bodies
— early degenerative arthritis.

■ *Failed previous shoulder surgery*: With patients whose symptoms persist after open shoulder surgery, the first factor to be considered is whether the original diagnosis was correct. As discussed, Cofield's work[1] makes clear that clinical diagnosis is an unpredictable art. For this reason, shoulder arthroscopy can be useful. Diagnosis may be changed or confirmed, or a second pathology revealed.

However, assessment of the rotator cuff can be very difficult after previous open surgery. For example, the arthroscopist may be misled when thin scar tissue gives the impression that the cuff is intact, although mechanically the cuff behaves as if it were disrupted. Cuff function is dependent on a good mechanical reconstruction with full thickness cuff material. Furthermore, adhesions may develop in the subacromial bursa, making visualization of the cuff repair difficult (Figure I).

Other areas where symptoms may remain following open surgery are unrecognized loose bodies, labral tears and early degenerative arthritis.

Arthroscopic surgery

During the latter half of the 1980s it became rapidly apparent that arthroscopy could not only be used as a diagnostic aid around the shoulder, but that it could be used therapeutically.

Immediately a philosophical enigma arose, namely that if arthroscopic surgery was more difficult and less successful than open surgery, then how could it be justified? Avoidance of scar tissue and speed of recovery seemed to be given more emphasis than the efficacy of treatment and the long-term outcome. Added to this was the problem that patients started to vote with their feet, for they had seen how successful minimally invasive surgery had been in the knee, and wanted their shoulder surgery performed by what the media labelled 'painless, bloodless surgery'.

We have subdivided the plethora of arthroscopic surgical procedures into five generations of increasing complexity (see page 125). Generally the earlier generations of surgery are technically easier and the results are better. Removal of loose bodies and trimming of labral tears are in generation one. Both of these procedures are relatively easy to carry out and can give significant benefit to the patient, with minimal risk of morbidity.

The best of the second generation procedures is arthroscopic subacromial decompression (ASD) (Chapter 8). The medium-term results of this type of surgery in experienced hands is excellent and its popularity will increase in the next five years. However, it is technically difficult with a long learning curve.

The third and fourth generations of arthroscopic surgery are forms of anterior reconstruction and complex reconstruction of traumatic instabilities (Chapter 9). The five-year results from the pioneering centres are just becoming available and these show 80–90 per cent short-term success rates[4]. Since these results are from the best centres, by the most skilled surgeons using the most up-to-date equipment, in a concentrated practice, then it is unlikely that the occasional arthroscopic shoulder surgeon will be able to achieve anything like such good results. This should be compared with the 90–95 per cent long-term success rates of open repair techniques such as the Bankart repair, and the Magnusson Stack procedure.

Arthroscopic repair, however, has a shorter learning curve than ASD. The arthroscopic views far exceed the view at open surgery and, in many ways, the procedure is 'easier' than the open procedure, which is technically demanding. This is the area of surgery of most rapid change and evolution and it would be wise for the inexperienced to avoid these procedures until further data is recovered from prospective controlled studies. Whether this advice can hold back the tide of patients who will demand this type of surgery, history alone can tell.

The final and fifth generation of arthroscopic surgery includes rotator cuff repair. There is a place for the arthroscopic repair of small rotator cuff tears at present. This can be carried out either with small arthroscopic suturing instruments under vision, or by using arthroscopic staples which are retrieved arthroscopically at six weeks, so as not to cause any damage to the undersurface of the acromion.

Arthroscopic debridement for massive rotator cuff tears is stated to relieve pain, although of course it cannot increase shoulder function. Acceptable results are not presently reproducible, and again this type of surgery should only be performed as part of a prospective controlled series, the patient having undergone informed consent as to the unpredictable nature of the results.

It has to be said that there is increasing concern expressed by all shoulder surgeons about the insertion of metal around the shoulder joint. Metal implants of all types (staples and screws) are known to move frequently from their initial position if placed around the shoulder. Presumably this occurs because of the shoulder's large range of motion and the excessive forces which will occur as a consequence on these metal implants. The shoulder also seems to attract metal implants, and once metal enters the shoulder joint it can lead to rapid and devastating loss of the articular surface. In order to circumvent this problem, biodegradable staples are currently being tested.

Naturally, arthroscopic surgery should not be attempted without adequate training. Hopefully this and other books will be a good starting point for surgeons in training, or for surgeons who want to develop the techniques of diagnostic shoulder arthroscopy. The next stage is to attend a shoulder arthroscopy course and then to work with an experienced shoulder arthroscopic surgeon. Only after performing some 50 diagnostic arthroscopies should the aspiring shoulder arthroscopist attempt the more simple 'first generation' techniques. Second generation surgery should only be undertaken after 100 diagnostic arthroscopies have been performed, and presently third generation surgery and upwards should only be performed by skilled shoulder arthroscopists as part of prospective controlled studies.

Finally, it must be remembered, that arthroscopy alone may help the patient but it is not a cure. Most cures for the shoulder still require the skills of open shoulder surgery and it must be stressed that shoulder arthroscopy should not be used unless the surgeon has, or develops, the skills of open shoulder surgery. Over the last few years, minimally invasive surgery of the shoulder using the arthroscope has begun to show promise. Just as arthroscopic meniscectomy popularized the use of the arthroscope in the knee, this ability to treat shoulder disorders arthroscopically may well drive shoulder arthroscopy in the coming years. For this reason, we have included three chapters on arthroscopic surgery of the shoulder, while realizing that this is such a rapidly changing field that methods outlined in this book will inevitably be replaced by even better techniques in years to come.

1 Extracapsular anatomy for shoulder arthroscopy

Introduction

The shoulder is the root of the upper limb. Because of this, the anatomy surrounding the joint is much more complex than the knee, and the hazards correspondingly greater for the arthroscopist. The knee is a simple joint to arthroscope as the soft tissue envelope around it is thin, the joint space can easily be felt, and landmarks are simple to distinguish. There are only two hazards: the neurovascular bundle and the lateral popliteal nerve, helpfully located far from the usual portal sites. This should be contrasted with the shoulder which has a thick, soft tissue envelope, where the joint space cannot be felt, landmarks may be difficult to distinguish, particularly in obese or muscular patients, and the joint is surrounded by six major nerves – the axillary artery, and five of its six branches, as well as the cephalic vein. Thus, not only is the anatomy more complex but major nerves are situated only millimetres from the two major portals. The suprascapular nerve passes 1 cm from the posterior joint line, and the musculocutaneous nerve enters the coracobrachialis directly in front of the anterior joint line. Nerve injury to the brachial plexus,[1] the musculocutaneous nerve[2] and the median nerve[3] have all been reported. For these reasons, an intimate knowledge of gross shoulder anatomy is an absolute prerequisite to the aspiring shoulder arthroscopist.

Various dissections of the shoulder may be performed in order to examine the relationship of the nerves and vessels to the normal arthroscopic portals. This chapter is based on such observations.

Posterior portal

Figure 1.1 shows the muscular anatomy of the right shoulder, as seen from behind. The only constant and useful landmark is the posterior angle of the acromion. The posterior portal is placed 2 cm inferior and medial to this constant point (Figures 1.2 and 1.3).[4–7] The first muscle layer that the arthroscope will traverse is the deltoid muscle (Figure 1.4). If the dissection is taken further so that deltoid is detached from the acromion and spine of the scapula, and folded forward (Figure 1.5), the next anatomical layer can be seen.

The first structure to note is the axillary nerve emerging, along with the posterior circumflex humeral vessels, from below teres minor. This neurovascular bundle is only 3 cm below the posterior portal (Figure 1.6), a point of great importance if a second, accessory posterior portal is made in order to perform arthroscopic surgery (for instance, the removal of loose bodies from the infraglenoid recess). The axillary nerve has a singularly inappropriate name,

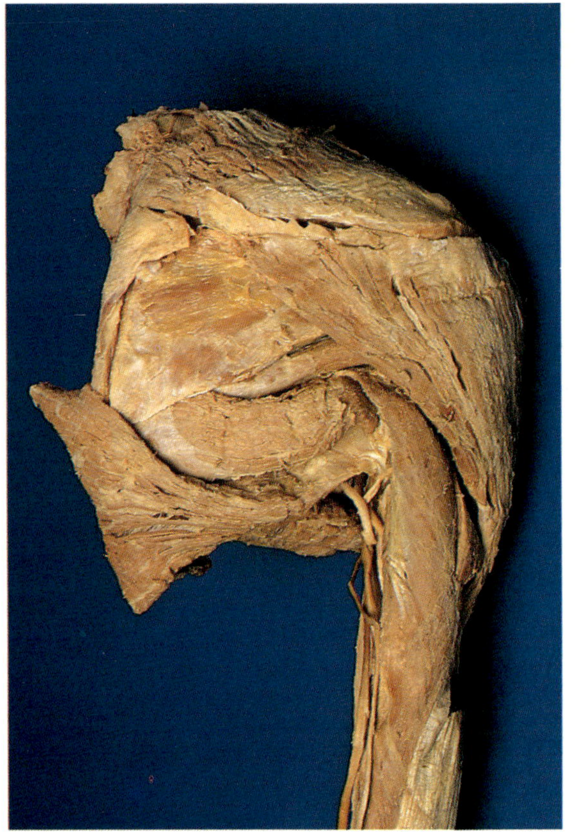

Figure 1.1

Muscular anatomy of the right shoulder seen from behind. The constant landmark is the posterior angle of the acromion, which you can feel on your own shoulder.

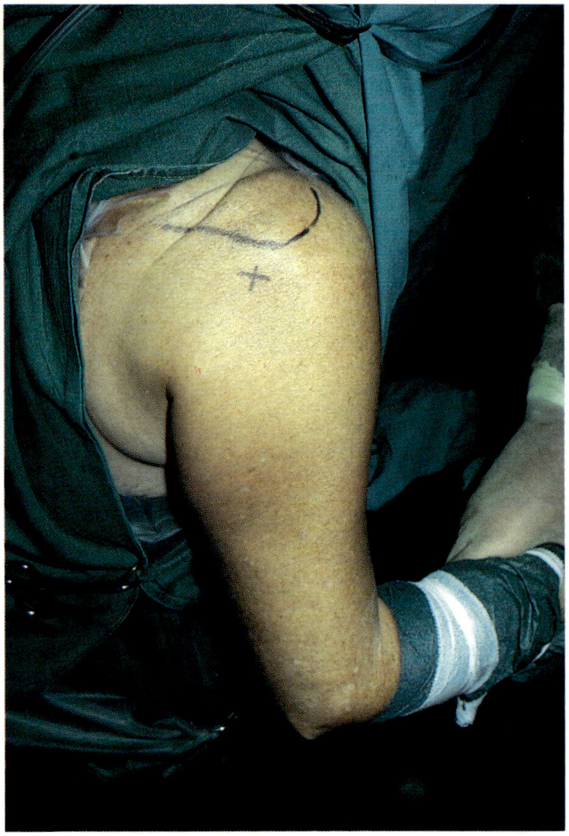

Figure 1.2

The posterior portal is situated 2 cm medial to and 2 cm inferior to the posterior angle of the acromion, as marked on this patient.

for the first thing it does on leaving the posterior cord of the brachial plexus is to pass below the inferior recess of the shoulder capsule and leave the axilla through the quadrilateral space. As can be seen, this is more a slit than a space, with teres major below, then the long head of triceps medially, humerus laterally, and finally teres minor above it.

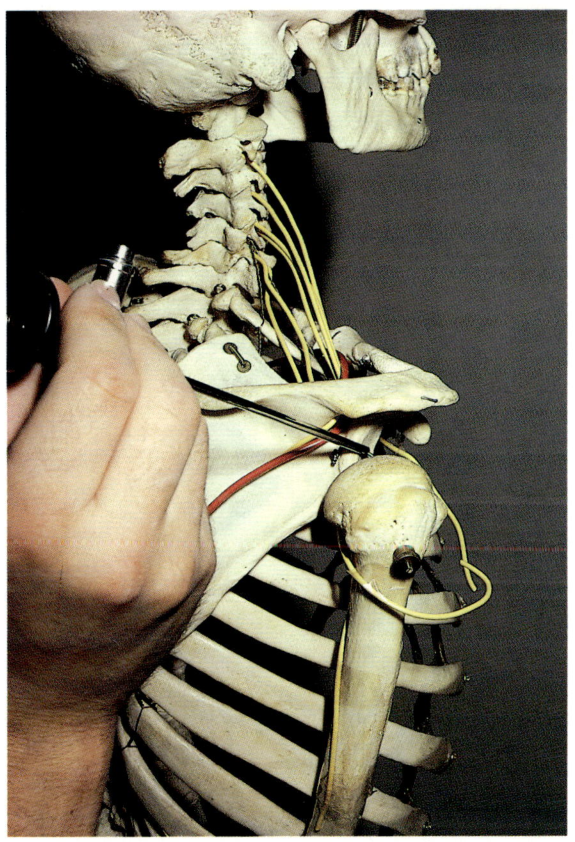

Figure 1.3

The posterior portal on the skeleton and the direction of the arthroscope entering the joint.

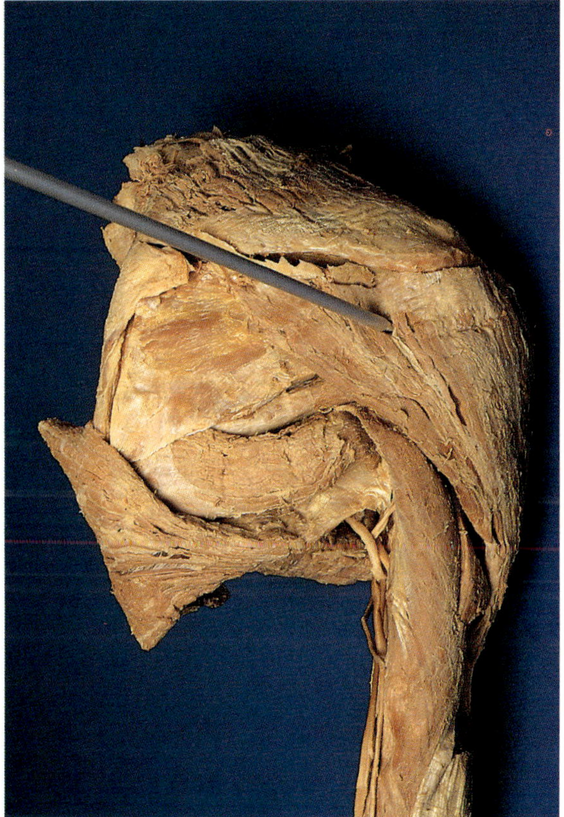

Figure 1.4

The arthroscope first passes through the posterior fibres of deltoid.

As the axillary nerve skirts the inferior border of the shoulder capsule it gives off branches to the joint, and divides into its two terminal branches, the deep and superficial branches. The superficial branch supplies teres minor and then appears behind the posterior border of deltoid to become the upper lateral cutaneous nerve of the arm (not shown on the dissection).

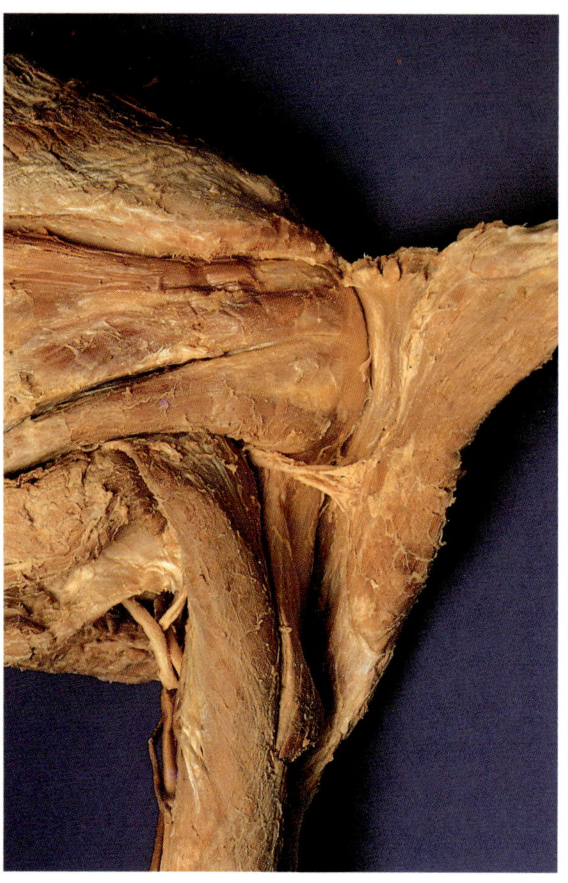

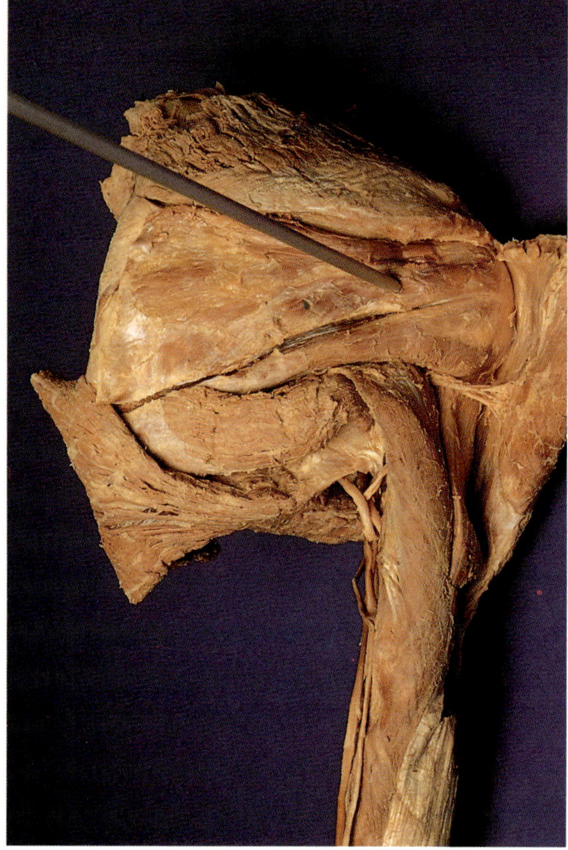

Figure 1.5

Deltoid is now retracted laterally, revealing infraspinatus and teres minor and their insertions into the humerus as the rotator cuff. Note the position of the axillary nerve and the posterior circumflex humeral vessels.

Figure 1.6

Note the distance of the axillary nerve from the arthroscope entering infraspinatus from the posterior portal.

The larger deep branch can be seen to divide and enter the deltoid muscle along with branches of the posterior circumflex humeral artery.

The next muscle layer that the arthroscope passes through is infraspinatus. In the next stage of dissection, infraspinatus has been lifted from its origin on the infraspinous fossa of the scapula, and folded up and outwards so that the track of the arthroscope can be clearly seen as it enters the joint (Figure 1.7), very close to the suprascapular nerve and artery. Branches of the suprascapular artery can be

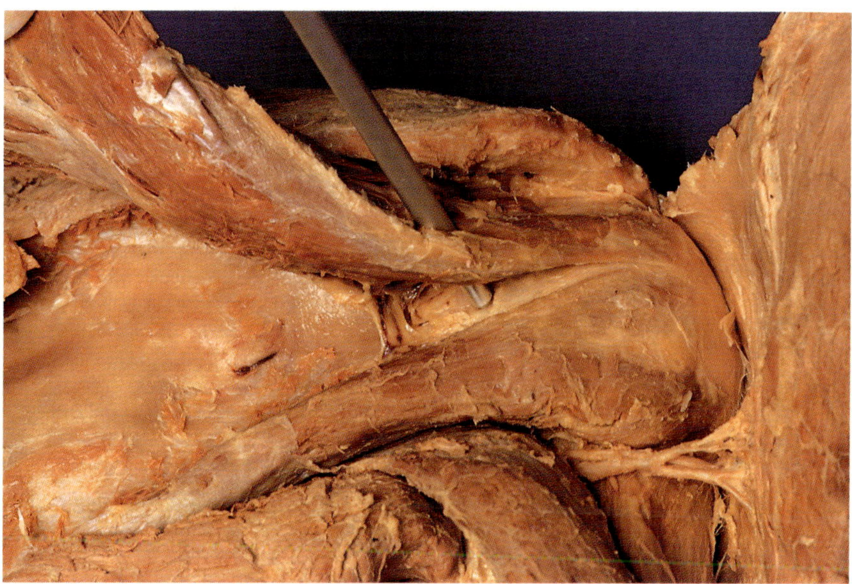

Figure 1.7

Infraspinatus has now been taken from its origin on the spine of the scapula and folded upwards to show the point of entry of the arthroscope through the posterior capsule of the shoulder joint. Note the close proximity of the ascending branch of the circumflex scapular artery (itself a branch of the subscapular artery), going to anastomose with the suprascapular artery.

seen passing downward, parallel to the joint line to anastomose with the circumflex scapular branch of the subscapular artery, in the scapular anastomosis. These vessels are obviously at risk if instruments are placed too far medially.

The suprascapular nerve is one of the most neglected of nerves and yet one of the most important to the shoulder. Mostly motor (it carries sensory and proprioceptive fibres from the glenohumeral and acromioclavicular joints, but contains no sensory fibres from skin), it leaves the upper trunk of the brachial plexus and runs a short course to the suprascapular notch, where it passes under the transverse ligament. Here its partner, the suprascapular artery, passes above the ligament. The nerve and artery then continue their journey, keeping close to the bone. The nerve supplies supraspinatus and passes around the base of the spine of the scapula (Figure 1.8) to supply infraspinatus. Thus the nerve is the motor supply to over one-half of the rotator cuff, and is as important to arm function as the femoral nerve is to leg function.

The next stage of the posterior dissection is to reflect the infraspinatus and the teres minor tendons medially, exposing the posterior capsule and to open the capsule close to the glenoid rim (Figure 1.9). The back of the humeral head can now be seen, along with the so-called 'bare area', or synovial reflection, which arthroscopically should not be confused with a Hill–Sachs lesion.

Finally the head of the humerus is osteoto-

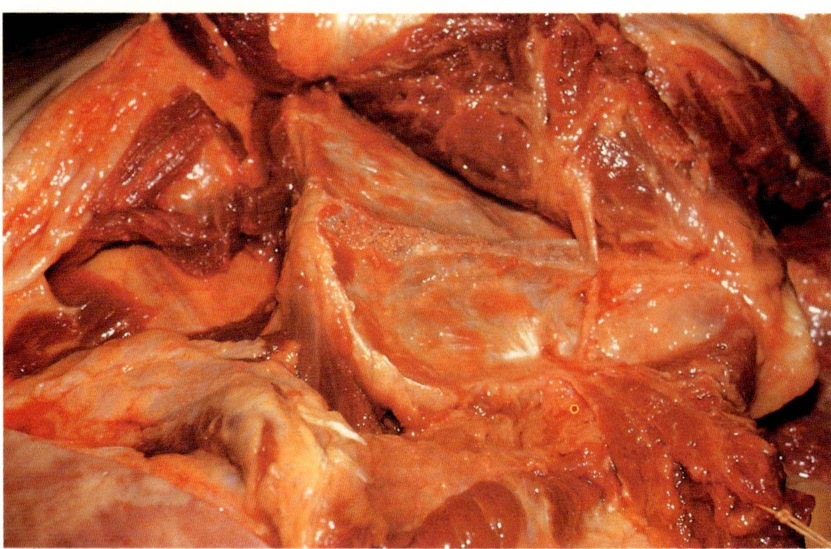

Figure 1.8

In this dissection, the spine of the acromion has been osteotomized and removed along with trapezius and deltoid. Supraspinatus and infraspinatus have then been lifted from their origins on the blade of the scapula to show the suprascapular nerve passing around the edge of the spine to supply both muscles.

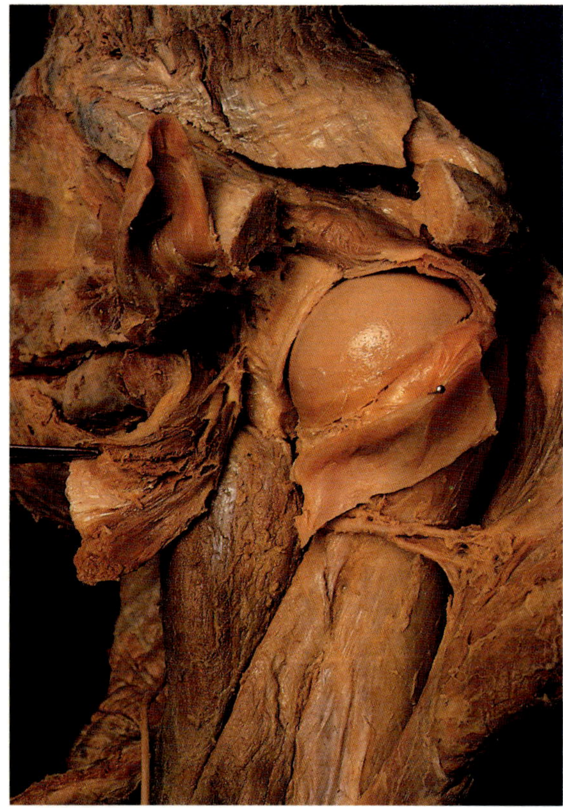

Figure 1.9

Infraspinatus and teres minor have now been reflected back and the posterior capsule of the shoulder has been incised at its origin from the neck of the glenoid and reflected laterally. The 'bare area' of the humeral head can be seen.

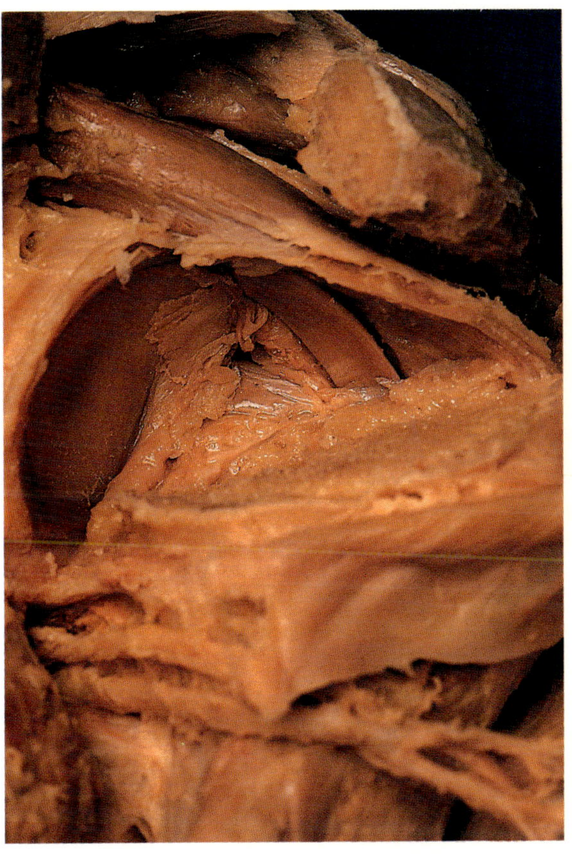

Figure 1.10

The head of the humerus has now been osteotomized and removed exposing the glenoid, the glenoid labrum, the long head of biceps and the anterior glenohumeral ligaments.

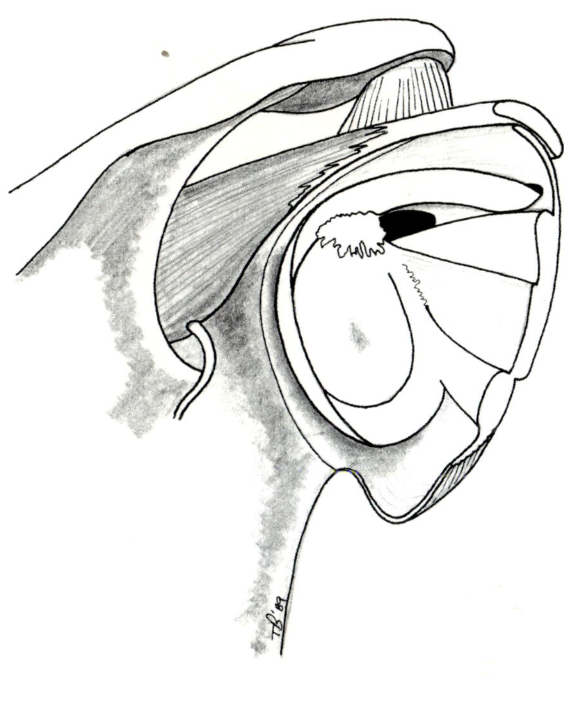

Figure 1.11

A simplified interpretation of the capsular structures as seen at arthroscopy.

mized to expose the anterior capsular structures arthroscopically (Figure 1.10). It is important at this stage to notice the close relationship of the axillary nerve and posterior circumflex artery as they pass directly under the inferior aspect of the joint. The glenoid can clearly be seen along with its central grey spot and surrounding labrum. The long head of biceps can be seen running across the top of the joint cavity, and below it the superior surface of the subscapularis tendon (Figure 1.11).

The anterior portal

Figure 1.12 shows the anterior aspect of the left shoulder. The deltopectoral groove can be seen, containing the cephalic vein. The anatomical landmarks for the anterior portal are the anterior acromion, the acromioclavicular (AC) joint and the tip of the coracoid process (Figures 1.13 and 1.14). Matthews[3] has shown how the anterior portal should be above and lateral to the tip of the coracoid process. In no circumstances should any instrument be placed inferior or medial to the coracoid process, as this would jeopardize the brachial plexus and the vascular supply of the whole upper limb. Figure 1.15 shows the position of the standard anterior portal which passes through deltoid and lateral to the cephalic vein.

Deltoid is now dissected free from its anterior origin on the clavicle and anterior border of the acromion. Pectoralis major is folded out laterally to expose the tendons of pectoralis minor and the conjoined tendons of coracobrachialis and short head of biceps originating from the coracoid process (Figure 1.16). The brachial plexus can be seen 5 cm below the coracoid. The musculocutaneous nerve leaves the lateral cord of the brachial plexus and enters the coracobrachialis muscle at a variable site 2–5 cm distal to the coracoid process. The musculocutaneous nerve supplies coracobrachialis and the short head of biceps as it passes through these muscles; it then supplies the rest of biceps and brachialis to emerge in the cubital fossa of the elbow as the lateral cutaneous nerve of the forearm.

The brachial plexus emerges from the axilla as three large mixed motor and sensory nerves (median, ulnar and radial) and two purely sensory nerves (medial cutaneous nerves of arm and forearm). The radial nerve is a continuation of the posterior cord and passes through the triangular space below teres major, with the humeral shaft laterally and the long head of triceps medially. The remaining nerves surround the axillary artery and vein and run on to the medial side of the arm.

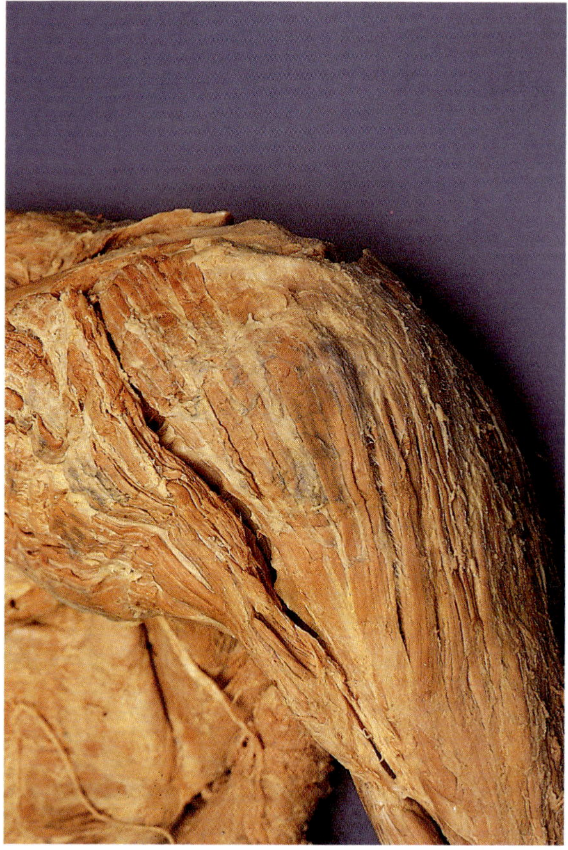

Figure 1.12

Muscular anatomy of the left shoulder seen from the front.

The axillary artery (Figures 1.17 and 1.18) has six branches. The first is the superior thoracic artery which leaves the upper third of the main artery to run forward and supply the pectoral muscles. The next two branches – the

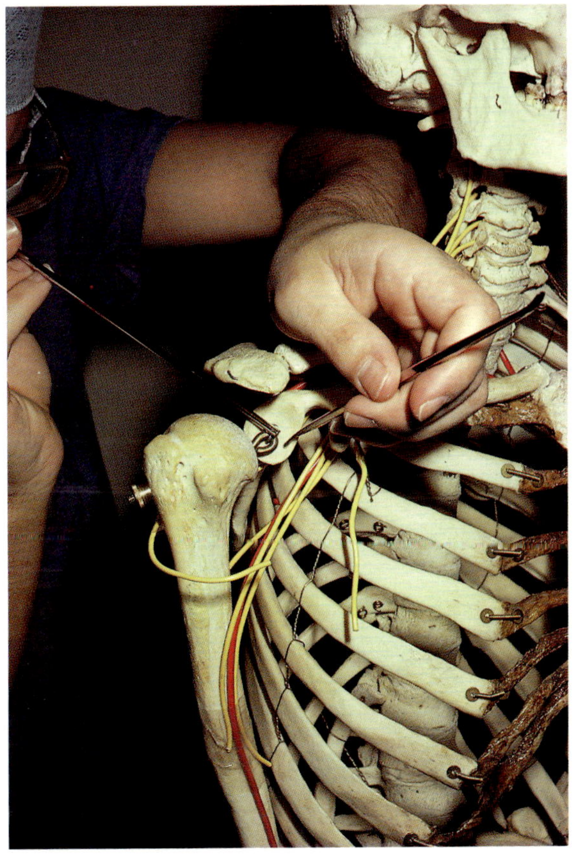

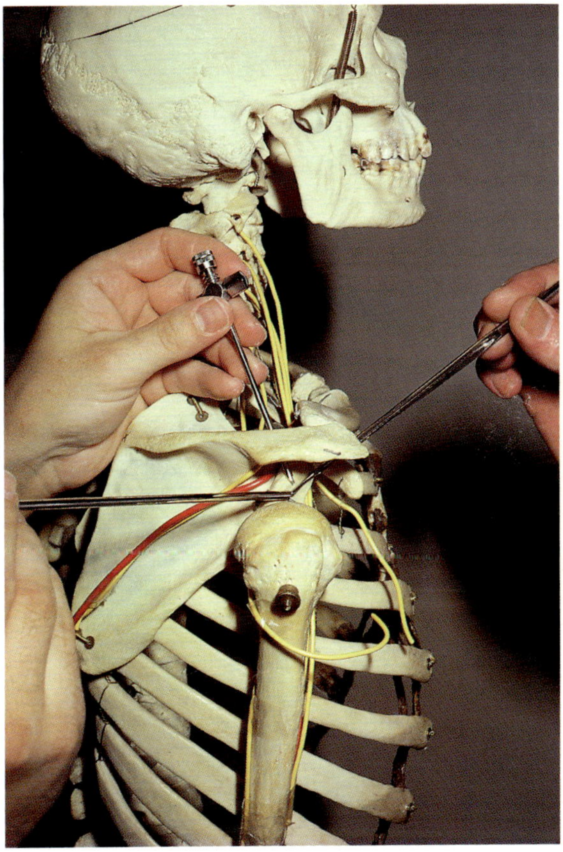

Figures 1.13 and 1.14

The anterior portal is made half way between the anterior edge of the acromion and the coracoid process, as shown on the skeleton.

Figure 1.14

acromiothoracic and lateral pectoral arteries – leave the middle third of the axillary artery as it passes under pectoralis minor. The acromiothoracic artery divides into four branches: the pectoral branches pierce the clavipectoral fascia and pass down to the muscle; the deltoid branch pierces the fascia and passes along within or under the deltoid paralleling the clavicle; and the acromial branch passes up alongside the coracoacromial ligament. The lateral thoracic artery passes down the chest wall on serratus anterior, supplying the pectoral muscles (and in women the breast).

The final three branches leave the third part

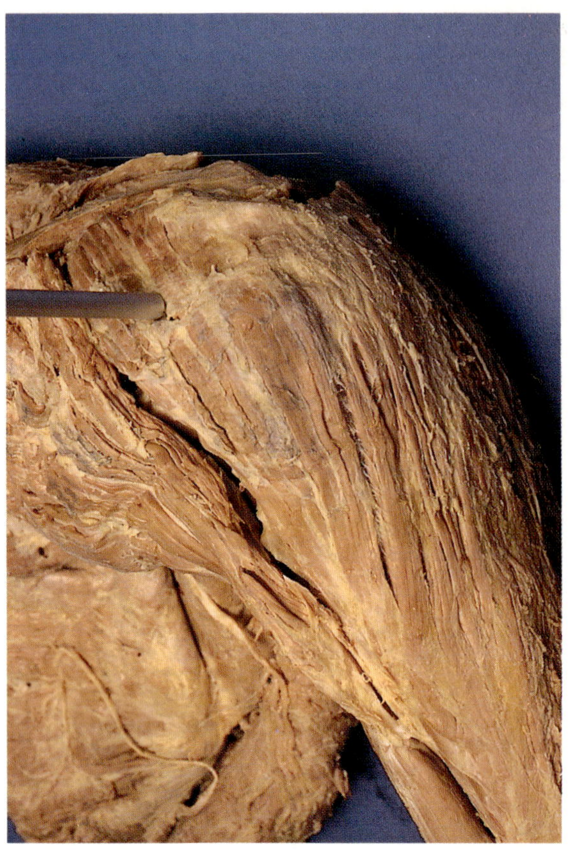

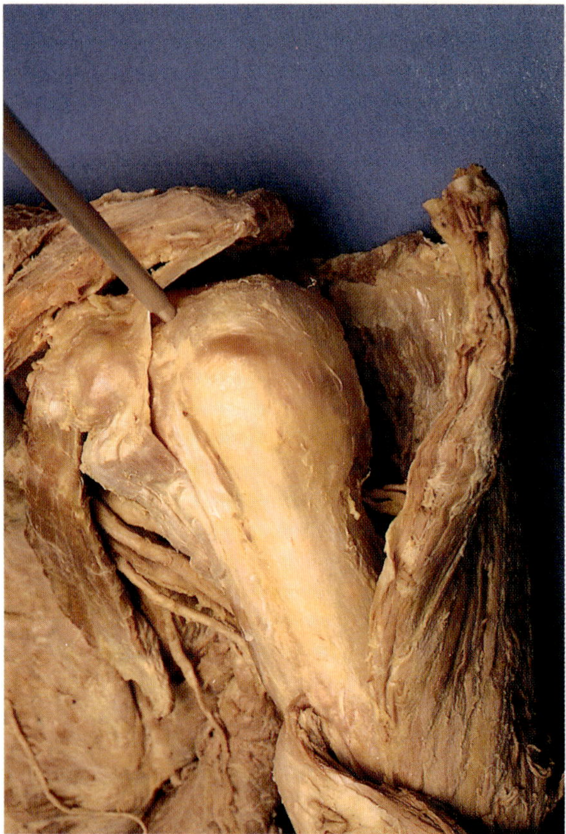

Figure 1.15

The arthroscope passes through the anterior deltoid, lateral to the cephalic vein.

Figure 1.16

The deltoid is now dissected from its origin on the acromion and folded laterally to show the path of the anterior portal. In this dissection, the arthroscope is shown passing the edge of the coracoacromial ligament. Usually, however, it passes through the ligament. Note the position of the brachial plexus.

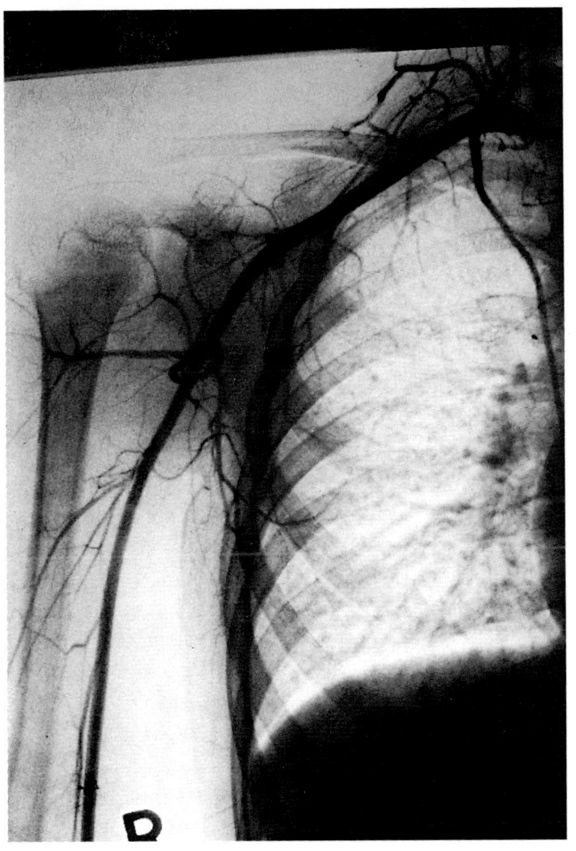

Figure 1.17

Arteriogram showing the major branches of the axillary artery.

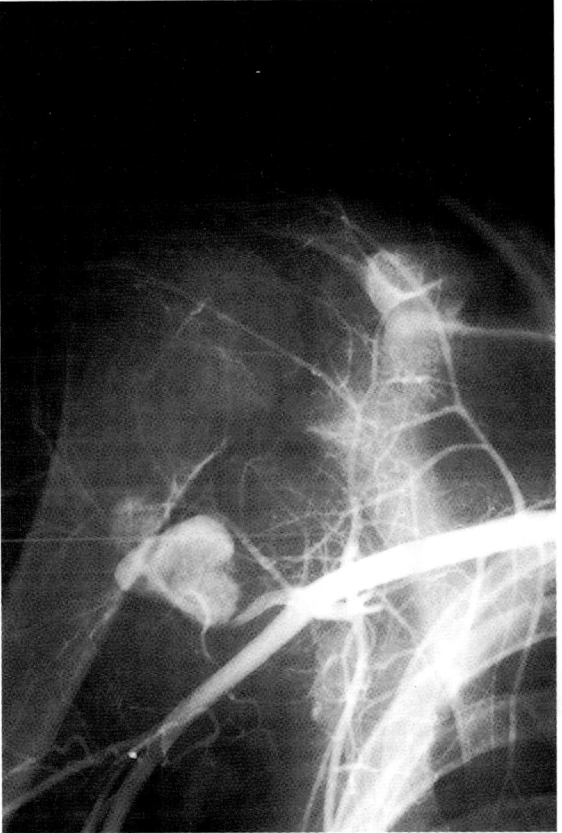

Figure 1.18

Arteriogram showing a close-up of the axillary artery. The patient had a traumatic false aneurysm of the posterior circumflex humeral artery.

of the axillary artery. The largest branch of this artery is the subscapular artery whose circumflex scapular branch anastomoses with the suprascapular artery. The anterior circumflex humeral artery runs along the inferior border of the subscapularis tendon to the humerus; here it gives an ascending branch which supplies the long head of biceps as it passes up the bicipital sulcus and goes on to supply the capsule and humeral head. The trunk of the anterior circumflex humeral artery passes around the humerus to anastomose with its larger partner, the posterior humeral circumflex artery, which has accompanied the axillary nerve through the quadrilateral space.

The coracoacromial ligament can be seen passing from coracoid to acromion. It is a large triangular ligament which inserts onto the undersurface of the anterior acromion, an important point to note when it comes to subacromial decompression. Having passed through deltoid, the instruments pass through the coracoacromial ligament or skirt its free edge to enter the joint just above the superior edge of the subscapularis muscle. Detrisac and Johnson[8] describe an occasional anterior capsular artery in close proximity to the superior glenohumeral ligament which can be damaged as the instrument traverses the anterior capsule at this point.

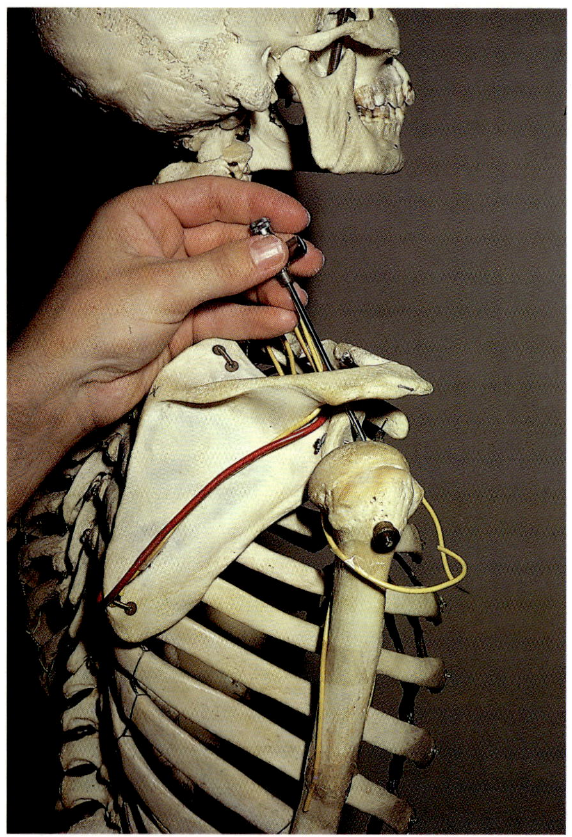

Figure 1.19

The superior portal: the needle is inserted medial to the acromion to enter the superior portion of the joint, as shown on the skeleton.

Superior portal

A superior portal has been described (Neviaser portal[9]) (Figure 1.19) which is useful for irrigating the shoulder joint. A needle is placed through the trapezius muscle, medial to the acromion, in the triangle bordered anteriorly by the clavicle and posteriorly by the spine of the scapula.

In the dissection, viewed from behind, trapezius has been dissected free from its insertion into the spine of the scapula and the acromion (Figure 1.20). The acromion has then been osteotomized from the spine of the scapula and tilted forward to expose the subacromial space. This portal has been criticized by some who say that the instruments damage the tendon of supraspinatus. Figure 1.21 shows this not to be

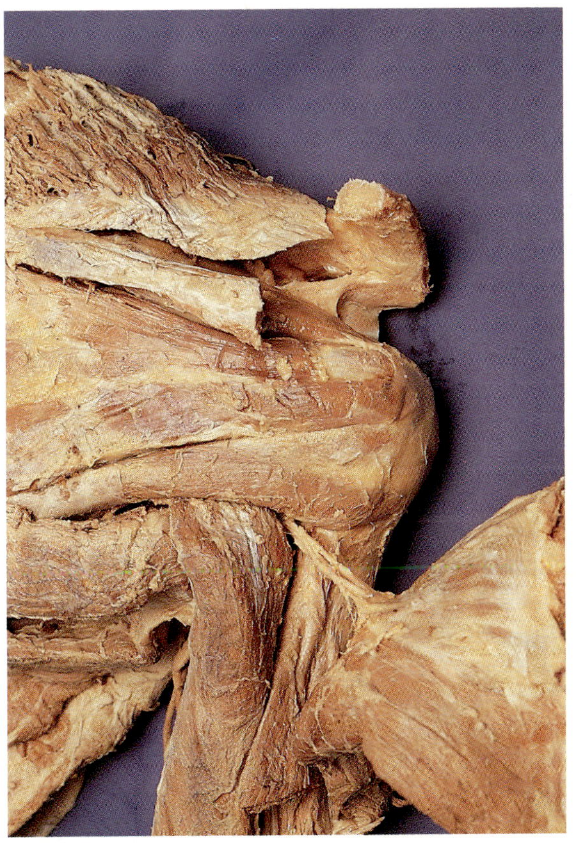

Figure 1.20

Trapezius has been dissected free and the acromion osteotomized to show the subacromial space.

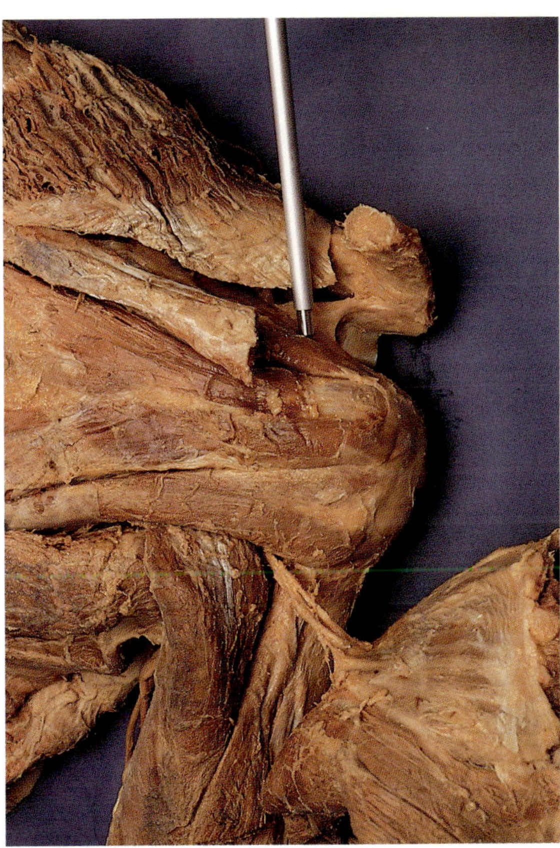

Figure 1.21

The arthroscope passes through the muscle fibres of supraspinatus.

the case – the instrument passes through the muscle fibres of supraspinatus, not the tendon, and this should not cause irreparable damage. The suprascapular artery and nerve are under the muscle at this point, about 2.5 cm medial to the portal.

Subacromial space

To the arthroscopic surgeon, the subacromial bursa is another cavity for exploration. This is helped by the fact that this is the largest bursa in the body and readily accepts 15 ml saline, just under half the capacity of the glenohumeral joint itself. Moreover the subacromial bursa is of particular interest to the shoulder surgeon since it is found at the impingement point, allowing the pathology of impingement to be seen. In fact the subacromial space is only a potential space, the bursa being two membranous surfaces separated by a thin film of lubricating fluid. It is only when the surgeon distends the bursa with irrigating fluid that a measurable space is created.

The first thing that the arthroscopic surgeon must understand is how far anterior the bursa is, for it is misnamed and should be called the subcoracoacromial ligament bursa. Figure 1.22 shows a dissection of the bursa which was prefilled with latex. As can be seen, the centre of the bursa is under the junction of the upper and middle thirds of the coracoacromial ligament, and the bursa hardly extends under the acromion at all. This is of vital importance to the arthroscopist, as the most common arthroscopic error is failure to enter the bursa, usually due to inability to visualize where the bursa ends.

Codman[10] dissected over 500 subacromial bursae and his detailed description is essential reading for arthroscopists. Prior to Codman's dissections, anatomists believed that there were separate subacromial, subdeltoid and subcoracoid bursae. Codman showed that these three were one, although sometimes the subacromial bursa could be partly loculated with plicae, just as the suprapatellar pouch may be subdivided by the suprapatellar plicae.

Strizak et al[11] found that three distinct components of the bursa could be identified in 15 dissections: subacromial, subdeltoid and subcoracoid. In 14 of these dissections, the subacromial and subdeltoid portions were confluent, but in one a septum separated the two portions. The subcoracoid portion was only identified in three dissections, extending more inferiorly and lying between subscapularis and coracoid, but never connecting with the glenohumeral joint.

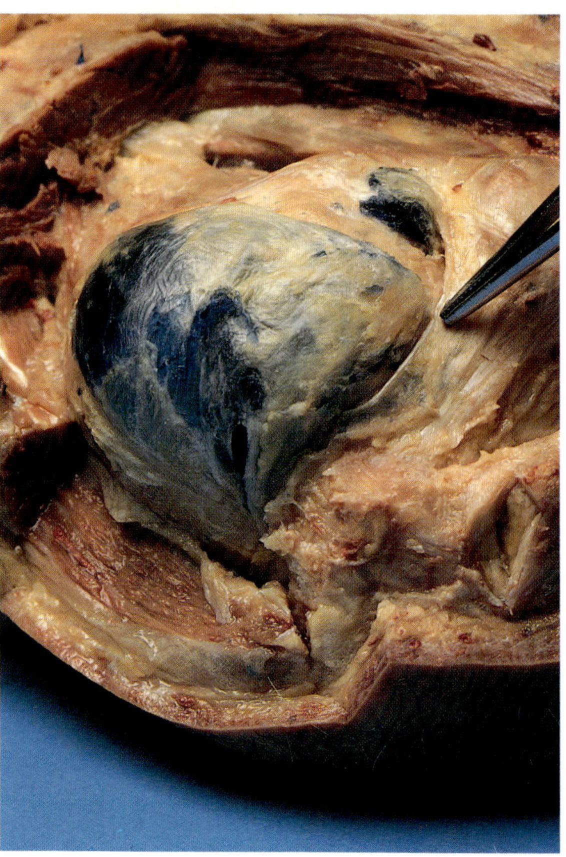

Figure 1.22

In this dissection of a left shoulder, seen from above, the subacromial bursa has been filled with blue gelatin. The forceps point to the centre of the free margin of the coracoacromial ligament. Note that the bursa hardly extends under the acromion at all.

The floor of the subacromial bursa consists of the tendon of insertion of supraspinatus, the shoulder capsule at the rotator interval, under which runs the tendon of the long head of biceps and the coracohumeral ligament. This corresponds to Laumann's middle zone of the subacromial space.[12]

The roof corresponds to the middle and upper thirds of the coracoacromial ligament,

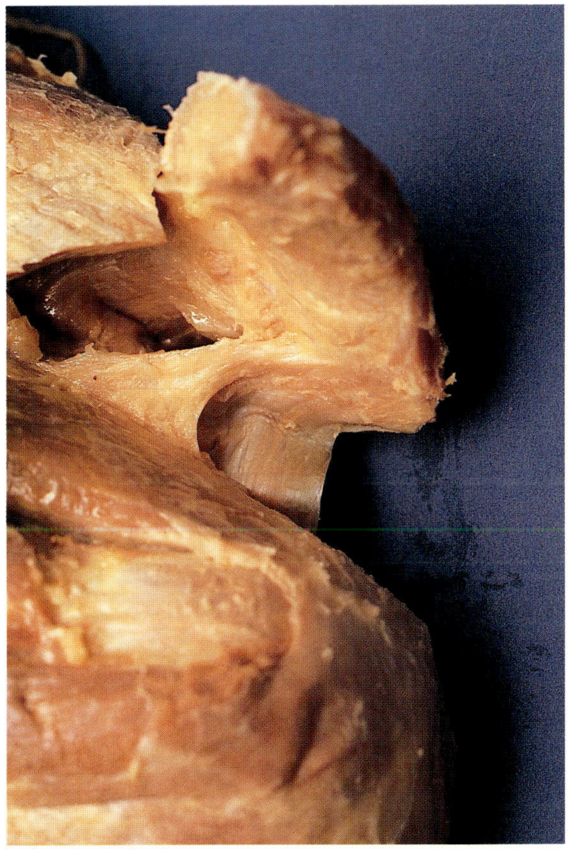

Figure 1.23

Note how the coracoacromial ligament inserts into the undersurface of the acromion.

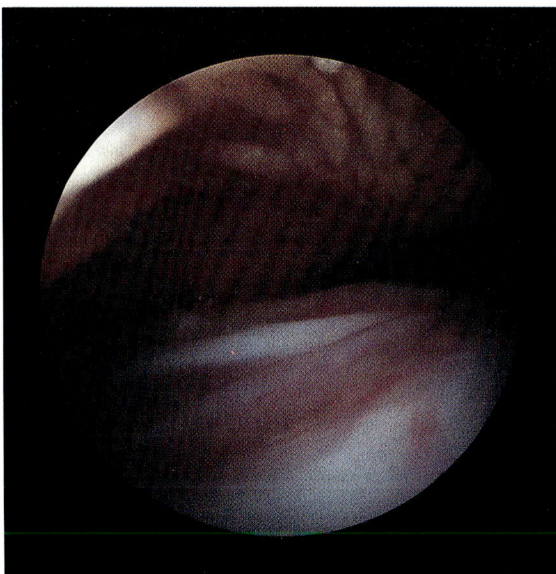

Figure 1.24

An arthroscopic view of the subacromial space showing the deltoid insertion.

the anterior third of the acromion and the undersurface of the acromioclavicular joint. It should be noted how the coracoacromial ligament inserts onto the undersurface of the anterior third of the acromion (Figure 1.23). Both the roof and the floor firmly adhere to these tissues.

The walls can only be described when the bursa is inflated, an unnatural condition. Moreover, if the bursa is inflated it changes shape from two flat surfaces in apposition to a sphere. As the height of the space increases, its diameter must decrease correspondingly, changing the position of the walls. Perhaps it would be better to call the walls the 'reflections' of the bursa. The lateral reflection is under the deltoid muscle (Figure 1.24)[11]; the posterior reflection, at the junction of the anterior and middle thirds of the acromion; the anterior reflection, under the coracoacromial ligament or, if a subcoracoid extension is present, under the coracoid; the medial reflection, under the acromioclavicular joint.

For more detailed descriptions, the reader should study the works of Codman,[10] Strizak,[11] Laumann[12] and Matthews et al.[13,14]

2 Assessment of the shoulder

History

Diagnosis of shoulder disorders depends mainly upon the history. There are often few signs to elicit. Patients will usually complain of either shoulder pain or loss of function. Rarer presentations may include instability, clicking, popping, snapping, a numb or 'dead arm', weakness or stiffness.

There are three key questions that need to be answered:

- Is this true shoulder pain?
- How did the pain start?
- Which movement exacerbates the pain?

Is this true shoulder pain?

True shoulder pain is felt at the shoulder and radiates into the upper arm. The patient will describe this in one of two ways. The palm sign describes the patient placing the palm of the unaffected hand over the epaulette area of the painful shoulder and rubbing. This is the usual presentation of glenohumeral or subacromial true shoulder pain (Figure 2.1). The finger sign describes the patient taking the index finger of the opposite hand and pointing to the affected acromioclavicular joint which is pathognomonic of acromioclavicular joint pain (Figure 2.2). True shoulder pain must be differentiated from neck pain, radicular pain and referred pain.

Neck pain originates in the neck and may be referred down to the shoulder, into the interscapular area or up towards the scalp. Root pain may be felt around the shoulder, but originates from the base of the neck and radiates all the way down the arm into the hand. Pain may be referred to the shoulder from diaphragmatic irritation, classically from gall-bladder disease to the right shoulder and from the heart to the left shoulder (Figure 2.3).

How did the pain start?

The patient may volunteer that the problem started with an injury. If so, a detailed description should be sought:

- When was the injury?
- What happened?
- Was it a soft tissue injury, a fracture or a dislocation?
- What was the position of the arm?
- How much energy was absorbed by the arm?
- How was it managed and by whom?
- Were radiographs taken?

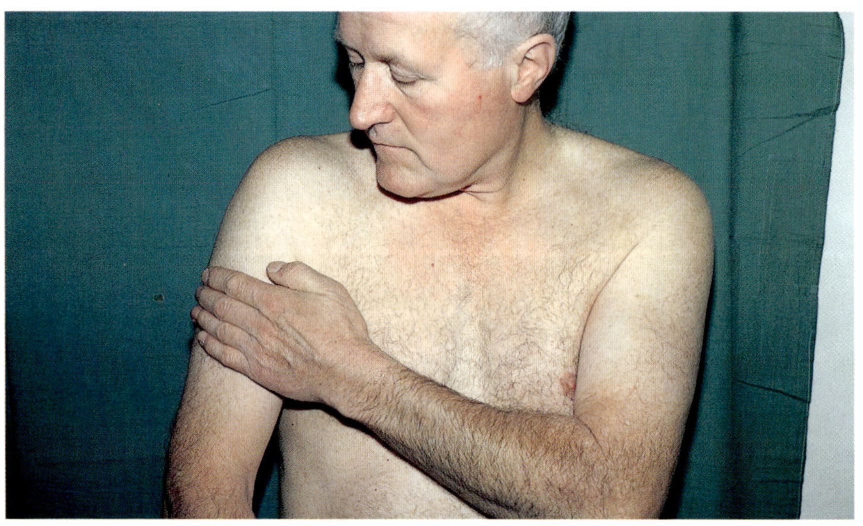

Figure 2.1

The 'palm sign': the patient points to the site of glenohumeral pain by rubbing the shoulder with the palm of the opposite hand.

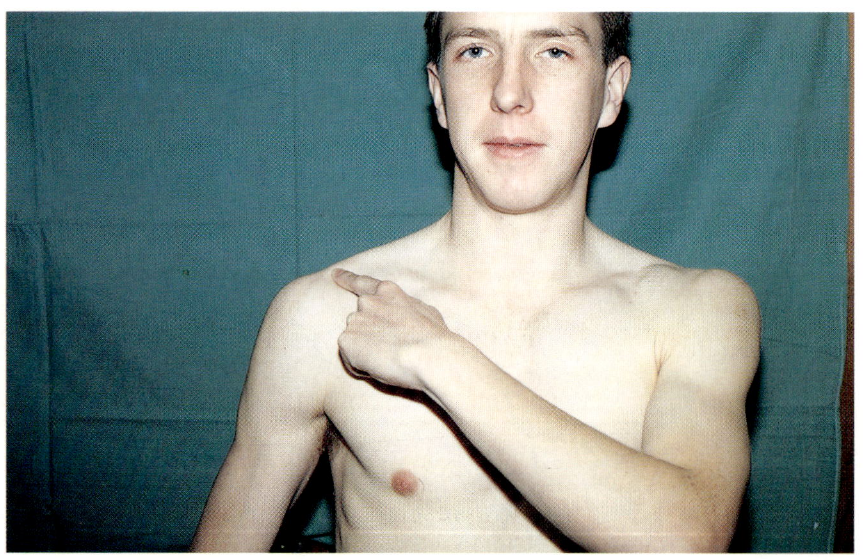

Figure 2.2

The 'finger sign': the patient points to the acromioclavicular joint pain with one finger directly on the affected joint.

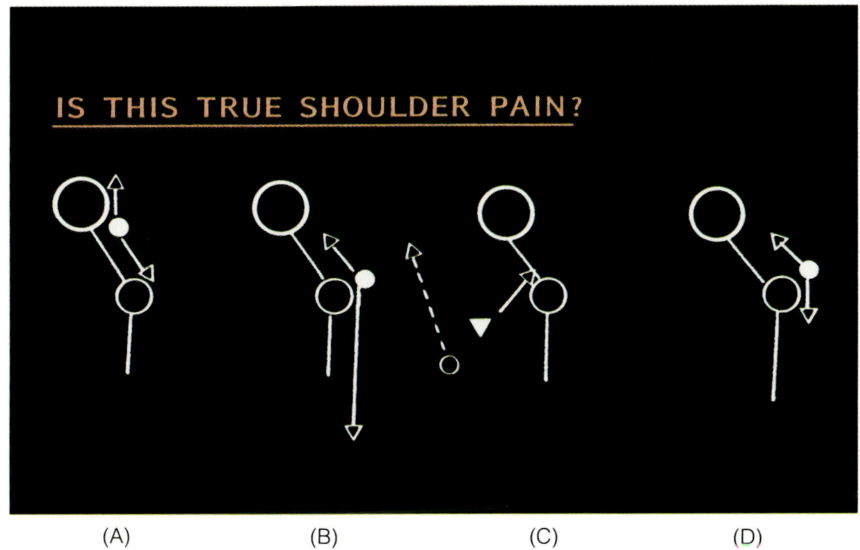

(A) (B) (C) (D)

Figure 2.3

Types of shoulder pain. From left to right: neck pain starts at the neck and radiates to the shoulder and up into the scalp (A). Root pain may be maximal at the shoulder but radiates down the length of the arm to the hand (B). Pain may be referred to the shoulder, classically from the diaphragm and gallbladder to the right shoulder and from the heart to the left shoulder (C). True glenohumeral joint pain may radiate both down the arm and also, to a lesser extent, up into the neck (D).

— To what degree did it recover and in what time period?

If there was no injury:

— Did the pain come on suddenly or insidiously?
— Is there any history of arthritis in any other joint?
— Has the patient had any recent infections?
— Is the patient generally well?

Which movement exacerbates the pain?

Pain at rest is a worrying symptom. The patient may be systemically unwell or well. If the patient is systemically unwell, then sepsis or polymyalgia rheumatica should be considered. If the patient is well, then the pain is usually due to early arthritis of the shoulder or a developing capsulitis (frozen shoulder). These patients will usually have a stiff shoulder on examination with limitation of external rotation and limited flexion and abduction. They may have a terminal painful arc such that elevation is restricted to 100 degrees, with a painful arc between 70 and 100 degrees.

Pain on movement denotes a painful arc of which there are four types: terminal, of the stiff shoulder (capsulitis arc, as above); subacromial; acromioclavicular; and composite (Figure 2.4).

The *subacromial painful arc* produces an arc of pain which comes on at approximately 70 degrees of elevation or abduction and eases off at approximately 130 degrees to top elevation. This usually indicates pain arising from subacromial impingement. A trap for the unwary is that subacromial impingement in a patient under the age of 40 is often a sign of shoulder instability causing functional impingement (see Chapters 8 and 9). Proof of the pain originating in the subacromial region can be demonstrated by the impingement test (see below).

The *acromioclavicular painful arc* produces an arc of pain at the extreme of shoulder elevation, between 140 and 170 degrees. This usually denotes pain arising from the acromioclavicular joint which can be blocked by the injection of local anaesthetic.

The *composite painful arc* has a near normal

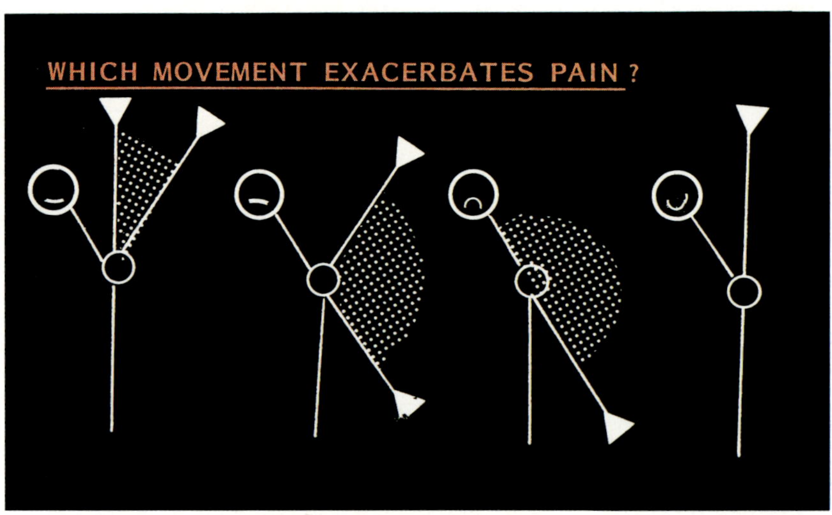

Figure 2.4

Which movement exacerbates the pain? From left to right: the high painful arc of acromioclavicular joint disease, the common painful arc of impingement, the stiff painful shoulder (frozen shoulder). Some people may have shoulder pain which is not exacerbated by movement.

range of shoulder elevation, but a painful arc from 70 degrees to the top of elevation, a fairly common situation. It occurs in patients with dual pathologies, such as acromioclavicular pain and subacromial impingement.

Severity of pain and function

Once the three key questions have been answered, the surgeon will gain further insight by enquiring into the severity of the pain, its frequency, pain at night (a particular feature of shoulder pain) and functional loss. The patient attending the shoulder clinic may be asked to complete a self-assessment sheet while waiting to see the surgeon (Figure 2.5). This scores pain from nil to severe (1–5), the frequency of pain from none to constant rest pain (1–5), and pain at night from none to unable to sleep every night (1–5). Thus a patient scoring 5s all the way is in severe trouble and is asked to complete a form on each attendance giving an objective assessment of improvement. The patient also marks on the form which movements make the pain worse and any change since the last attendance (better or worse). The surgeon also scores the pain and notes analgesic consumption on a separate assessment sheet (Figure 2.6).

Functional loss is as vital to the patient as pain and this is also scored on the self-assessment form. Reach is assessed to shoulder blades, shelves above head, hair, waist, back of neck, base of spine and opposite axilla. Finally, loss of work, sport and sleep are scored. Functional loss has been used by many surgeons who have tried to devise shoulder scoring systems. The Mayo score includes driving, dressing, sleeping and overhead working; the Neer score emphasizes perineal care, dressing, carrying, throwing and lifting. The Lysholm score is used in Sweden and the Constant score in the United Kingdom. Functional assessment based on the Neer score is included in the computerized diagnosis program used by Johnson, which is a 42-page document detailing medical history, shoulder history, shoulder examination, investigations, and shoulder surgery.

It is vital to know the patient's exact occupation and hand dominance and how this is affected by the shoulder pain, if this has not already been elicited at the start of the interview.

Specific questions

Specific questions may now be asked such as the presence of joint stiffness, clicking, popping or snapping sensations and jamming of the joint.

The patient should also be asked whether the joint has ever been dislocated. If so, the initial event should be documented, together with the number of recurrences, the direction of dislocation, the ease of reduction and any feelings of instability without the joint actually dislocating.

Examination

The examination really starts before the history is taken. For instance, a handshake may demonstrate the shoulder shrug of a full thickness massive rotator cuff tear (Figure 2.7). Particular attention should be paid to the difficulties the patient has in removing a shirt or jacket. The surgeon must remember that the shoulder is really a series of joints – the sternoclavicular, acromioclavicular, sternothoracic, subacromial and finally the glenohumeral. The neck should be examined, as should the elbow, wrist and hand. This chapter, however, will consider the shoulder girdle alone.

Examination consists of *look*, *feel*, *move* and *X-ray*.

PATIENT'S SELF ASSESSMENT SHEET: SHOULDER

NAME ....

SHOULDER AFFECTED: RIGHT/LEFT

TODAY'S DATE ....

SEVERITY OF PAIN
Choose one of the following by ringing the number.

1 I have no pain.
2 I have mild discomfort.
3 I have moderate pain which forces me to make concessions.
4 I have pain bad enough to need painkilling tablets.
5 I have severe pain.

FREQUENCY OF PAIN
Choose one of the following by ringing the number.

1 I have no pain.
2 I have occasional pain after unusual activity.
3 I have occasional pain on movement.
4 I have pain whenever I move my shoulder.
5 I have pain present all the time, even at rest.

PAIN AT NIGHT
Choose one of the following by ringing the number.

1 I have no pain at night.
2 My sleep is disturbed occasionally by pain in my shoulder.
3 I am woken at least once every night by pain in my shoulder.
4 I am woken several times each night by pain in my shoulder.
5 I am unable to get enough sleep every night because of pain in my shoulder.

PAINFUL MOVEMENTS
Ring all the numbers which apply to you.

1 Pain occurs when reaching behind my neck.
2 Pain occurs when reaching behind my waist.
3 Pain occurs when reaching above my head.
4 Pain occurs when reaching sideways.
5 Pain occurs when reaching forwards.

FUNCTIONAL LOSS
Ring which number is true when using your 'bad' arm.

1 I cannot reach between my shoulder blades.
2 I cannot reach a shelf above my head.
3 I cannot comb my hair.
4 I cannot reach behind my waist.
5 I cannot wash the back of my neck.
6 I cannot reach the base of my spine.
7 I cannot wash under the opposite arm.

1 I cannot do usual sport. (Name sport).
2 I cannot do usual work. (Name work).
3 I cannot sleep on that side at night.

CHANGE SINCE LAST ATTENDANCE
Compare your shoulder now with how it was when you last saw the doctor. Ring the number which best describes it.

1 My shoulder is much better.
2 My shoulder is a little better.
3 My shoulder is the same.
4 My shoulder is worse.

Figure 2.5

Sample shoulder assessment sheet (filled in by patient).

SHOULDER ASSESSMENT SHEET

One form to be completed for each shoulder.

Name .... DOB .... Diagnosis .... **L** or **R**

Address .... Hospital No. .... Previous treatment

Drug ....

Injection ....

Other ....

Surgery ....

Type of operation ....

Dominant hand R/L

Occupation .... Date ....

Surgeon ....

Other upper limb problems ....

OPERATION DATE (ring arrow) / Date (this assessment)		↓ 1st visit		↓ 2nd visit		↓ 3rd visit		↓ 4th visit		↓ 5th visit	
PAIN	At rest										
	On movement										
TAKING ANALGESICS	(yes/no)										
	Type										
	Number										
MUSCLE WASTING	Deltoid										
	Supraspinatus										
	Infraspinatus										
STRENGTH (S) + PAIN ON TEST (P)		S	P	S	P	S	P	S	P	S	P
	Abd										
	Flex										
	I rot										
	E rot										
RANGE OF MOTION (standing)		A	P	A	P	A	P	A	P	A	P
ACTIVE (A) +	Abd										
PASSIVE (P)	Flex										
	I rot										
	E rot										
	(Arm by side – segment covered by back of hand)										
	(Arm by side)										
CHANGE (since operation/treatment)											
ASSESSOR'S INITIALS:											
GRADE:											

PAIN ON REST OR MOVEMENT
0 = None
1 = Slight or occasional
2 = After unusual activity
3 = Moderate – alters use
4 = Marked – limits activity
5 = Severe – loss of sleep

WASTING
PAIN ON TEST (P)
0 = None
1 = Mild
2 = Moderate
3 = Severe

STRENGTH (S)
0 = Normal
1 = Mild weakness
2 = Severe weakness
3 = Paralysis

CHANGE
1 = Much better
2 = Better
3 = Same
4 = Worse

Figure 2.6

Sample shoulder assessment sheet (filled in by surgeon).

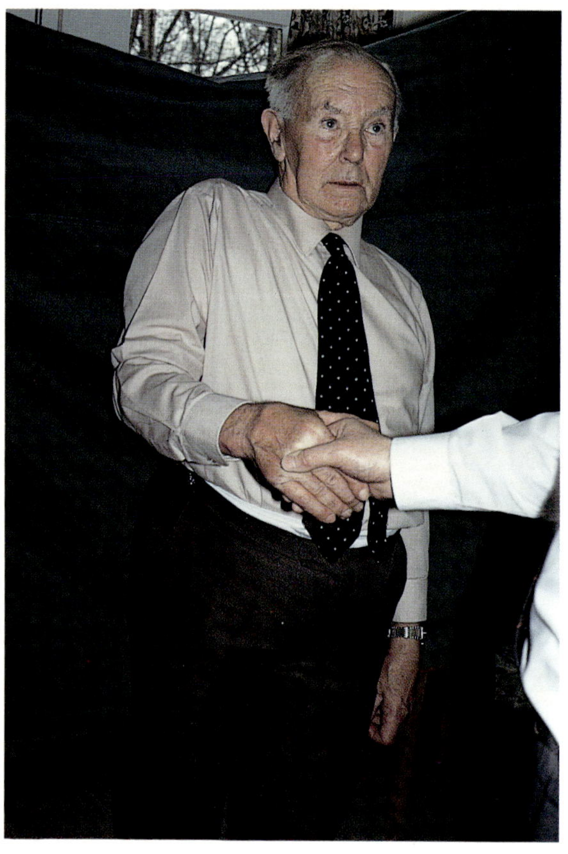

Figure 2.7

The shoulder shrug associated with a full thickness rotator cuff tear.

Look

Swelling, deformity or subluxation of the sternoclavicular, acromioclavicular or glenohumeral joints are noted, as are any swellings or deformity of the clavicle, humerus or scapula. The appearance of the skin is noted, and in particular any scars or incisions are inspected.

Muscle-wasting is of particular importance to the shoulder (Figures 2.8 and 2.9). The rotator cuff has been likened to the quadriceps, in that both have four muscle bellies (subscapularis, supraspinatus, infraspinatus and teres minor) and both waste rapidly with any abnormality of their associated joint. Wasting of supraspinatus and infraspinatus is easily seen and can be compared to the normal side. The thickness of the muscle and the tone in it can also be felt.

If wasting is extreme, then neuromuscular disease should be considered. Fascioscapulohumeral dystrophy often presents with loss of shoulder function, with marked proximal muscle wasting. Scapular winging may be the presentation of neuralgic amyotrophy. Marked and isolated wasting of supraspinatus and infraspinatus may point the way to a diagnosis of suprascapular nerve entrapment syndrome.

Feel

Palpation is of less value in the shoulder than in many other joints. Specific tenderness may be elicited on pressing over the sternoclavicular or acromioclavicular joints, but tenderness around the glenohumeral joint, hidden as it is under the cloak of the acromion and deltoid, is fairly unhelpful.

Subacromial crepitus, as the patient elevates the arm, can often be impressive, particularly in patients with rotator cuff tears. Some surgeons can feel the defect of a rotator cuff tear with the arm in an extended and adducted position when the impingement area of supraspinatus insertion is brought out from under the acromion, but this requires great experience.

Clicking or snapping should be felt in an attempt to locate the structure from which it emanates. A snapping scapula may be associated with osteochondroma of the blade of the scapula clunking over the ribs as the arm elevates. Clicking on instability testing or elevation may be due to subluxation or a labral tear.

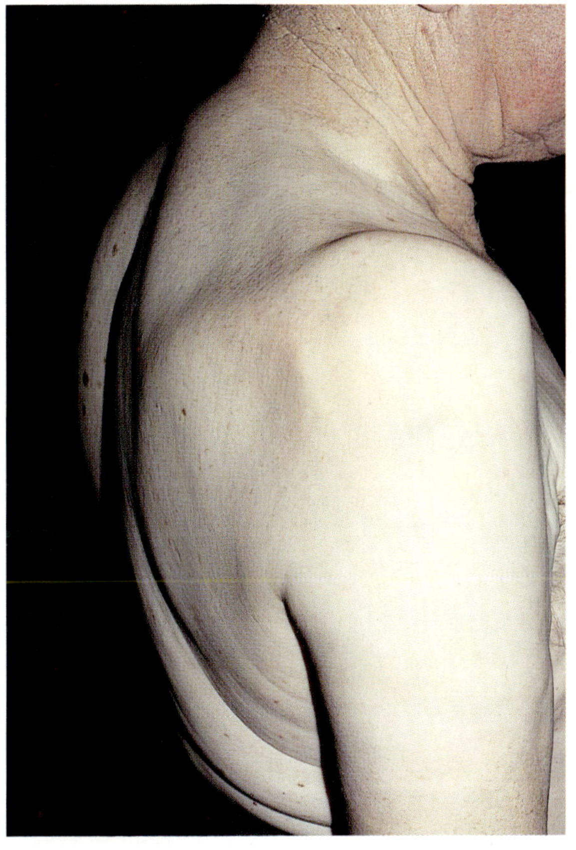

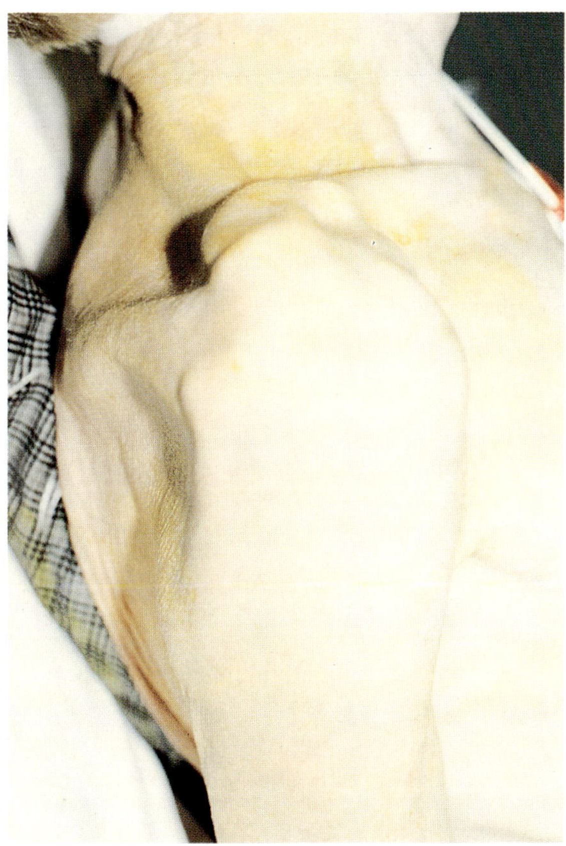

Figures 2.8 and 2.9

Wasting of the cuff muscles, moderate (2.8) and gross (2.9) following rotator cuff tears of long standing.

Figure 2.9

Move

Active movements

Active movements are assessed first. The patient is asked to elevate the shoulder to demonstrate any limitation of movement or painful arc. If movement is limited then an examining hand placed on the scapula during active elevation will show whether the limitation is glenohumeral or scapulothoracic, or both. A painful arc may be more marked with elevation in abduction rather than flexion. With the elbow locked into the side active external rotation is compared with the unaffected arm, and finally active internal rotation is assessed by comparing how far up the spine the thumb of the affected arm will go compared to the normal side. For this latter test, elbow function must be equal on both sides.

Passive movements

Elevation, external rotation and internal rotation are again measured with the surgeon holding the distal humerus in one hand and the inferior angle of the scapula under the palm of the other hand. The range, pattern of movement, end point, excess over active movement and degree of pain are all noted.

Rotator cuff strength

The clinical test of rotator cuff function is an integral part of every examination of the shoulder.

The supraspinatus test

This test (Figure 2.10) is carried out with the patient standing. With the elbow straight, the arm is placed in 20 degrees of abduction and flexion, and the patient is told to hold it there. The examiner assesses the strength of abduction, and the patient reports the amount of pain produced by this manoeuvre. The examiner then tests the opposite normal shoulder for comparison. Weakness on testing denotes a rotator cuff tear. Unfortunately, if there is a lot of pain, then weakness will be apparent due to pain inhibition, and the test will have to be performed after an impingement injection test.

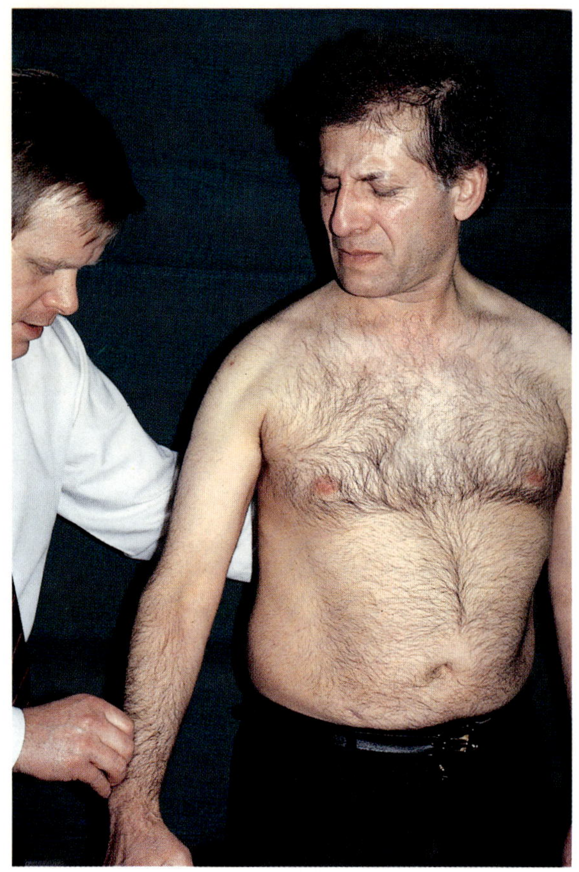

Figure 2.10
The supraspinatus test: active resisted abduction at 30 degrees tests supraspinatus strength.

The impingement injection test

This test allows the surgeon to establish whether subacromial impingement is causing the painful arc. For the test, 5 ml 1 per cent lignocaine (US: lidocaine) is injected under the anterior edge of the acromion. After 10 minutes the patient is re-examined, and if the painful arc is improved or abolished, then the site of pain has been established.

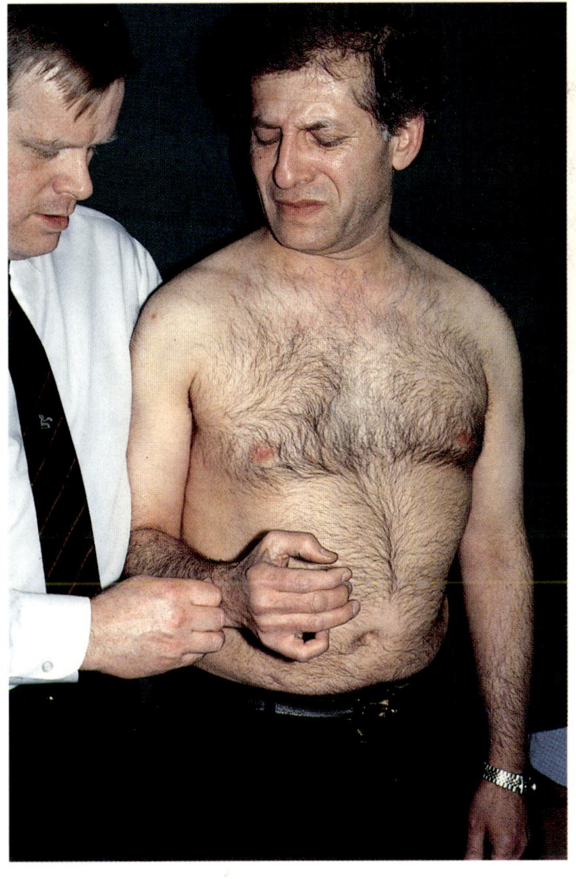

Figure 2.11

The infraspinatus test: active resisted external rotation with the elbow flexed to 90 degrees and the humerus at the side. Pain and weakness may denote a tear of infraspinatus.

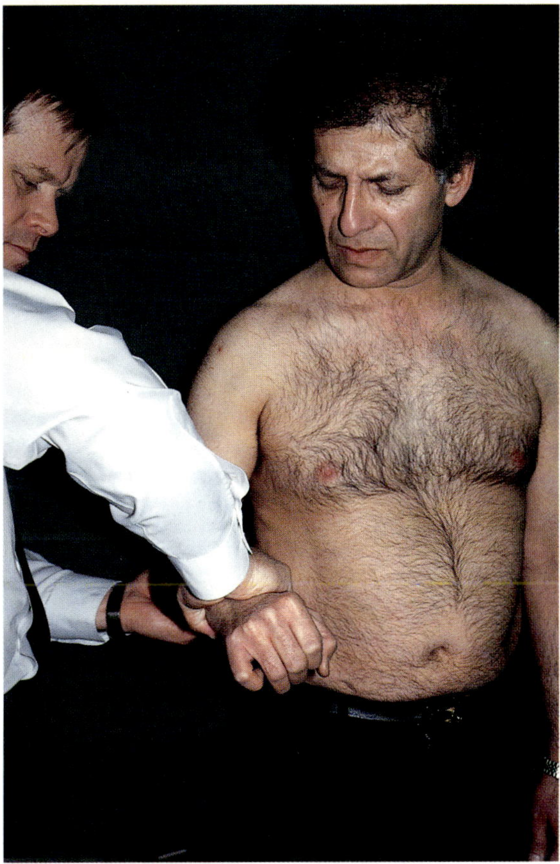

Figure 2.12

The subscapularis test: active resisted internal rotation of the glenohumeral joint.

The infraspinatus test

This test (Figure 2.11) is very similar to the supraspinatus test, and is a test of resisted active external rotation of the shoulder. The infraspinatus is the only efficient external rotator of the glenohumeral joint. Pain and weakness are sought, weakness denoting a rotator cuff tear.

The subscapularis test

This test (Figure 2.12) is similar, but opposite, to the infraspinatus test. With the elbow locked against the patient's side active resisted internal rotation of the glenohumeral joint is tested. Unfortunately this movement is produced by pectoralis major and latissimus dorsi, as well as subscapularis, and therefore is not such a sensitive test.

Special tests

Impingement tests

The impingement sign is produced by pushing the greater tuberosity upward against the inferior aspect of the acromion first in forward flexion, then in abduction and internal rotation, and finally in abduction and external rotation. [1,2] The tests are positive when painful and should be abolished with local anaesthetic under the anterior edge of the acromion.

Adduction test

Acromioclavicular joint pain is aggravated by forced adduction of the shoulder with the arm in 90 degrees of flexion (Figure 2.13). However, this test may also be painful in patients with subacromial impingement. An additional test is resisted active adduction of the shoulder with the arm hanging close to the side (Figure 2.14). Further evidence of acromioclavicular dysfunction can be obtained by repeating the tests after injection of 1–2 ml 1 per cent lignocaine (US: lidocaine) into the acromioclavicular joint.

Instability tests

These tests are essential in any patient under the age of 40 with shoulder pain, and should be performed not only in the outpatient office but before *every* shoulder arthroscopy when the patient is anaesthetized and fully relaxed.

Anterior apprehension test

The patient is examined sitting (or if anaesthetized, prior to arthroscopy, supine). The problem shoulder is passively abducted to 90 degrees, and is then passively externally rotated by the examiner into full external rotation. The arm is then pushed into the fully stressed position, while the patient's face is studied for apprehension. The normal shoulder is examined for comparison.

Shift and load test

Under anaesthesia, the shoulder is brought into the 'position of apprehension' and forcefully stressed to provoke subluxation or frank dislocation. Axial load is then applied down the humeral shaft onto the glenoid, and the abducted arm is brought forward into the flexed position, which puts a posterior shear force on the humeral head. If the humeral head had subluxed in the apprehension position then the 'load and shift' test will give a clunk as the shoulder relocates in a similar manner to the Ortolani test in congenital dislocation of the hip (CDH).

Anterior drawer test

To examine the right shoulder, the surgeon stands behind the seated patient, grasps the shoulder girdle with his left hand, the fingers at the front holding the clavicle and coracoid, and the thumb locked over the back of the spine of the scapula. The right hand then grasps the proximal humerus and forcefully translates the humerus forwards and backwards. Excess laxity is judged against the opposite side.

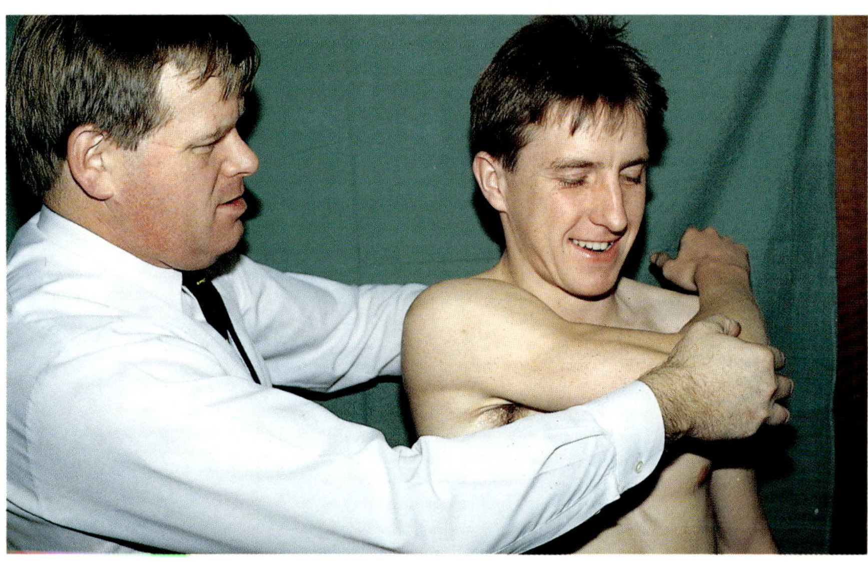

Figure 2.13
Acromioclavicular joint pain is aggravated by adduction of the shoulder with the arm in 90 degrees of flexion.

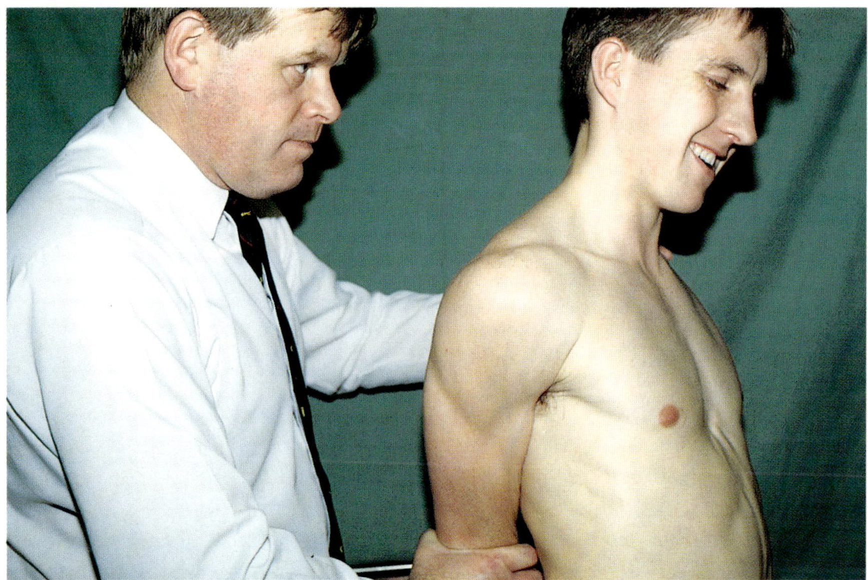

Figure 2.14
Acromioclavicular joint pain may also be found by adduction in extension.

The sulcus sign

The patient (usually a female, as this is a test for multidirectional instability) is seated with her arms hanging down on either side of the chair and asked to relax. The examiner applies downward traction on the arm by holding the wrist and distracting the arm downwards firmly but not roughly. If the shoulder is inferiorly unstable, a sulcus will appear between the acromion and the humeral head (Figure 2.15). This sulcus is both visible and palpable. The patient with a positive sulcus sign should be examined for generalized joint laxity.

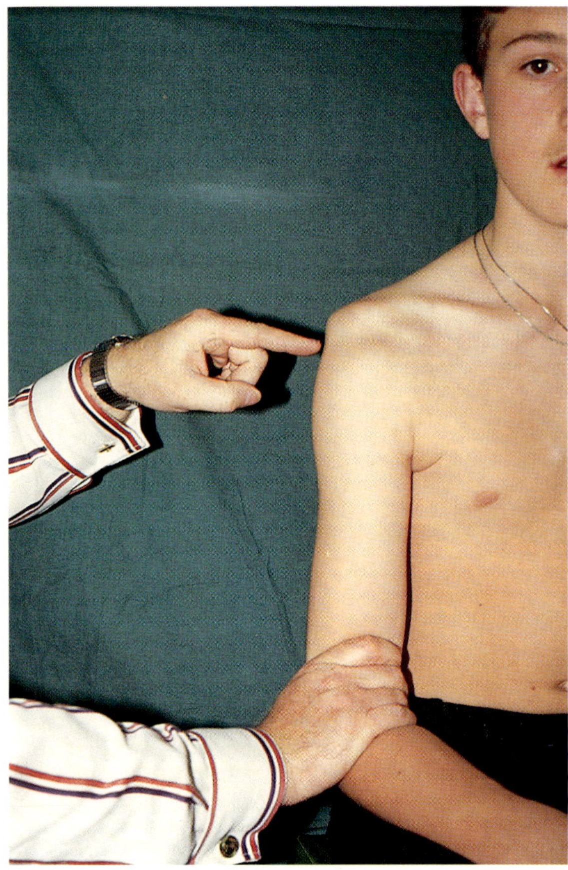

Figure 2.15

The sulcus sign: inferior traction on the arm in patients with multidirectional instability leads to the appearance of a sulcus between the acromion and the head of the humerus.

Posterior stress test

The patient is examined lying supine (Figure 2.16). The arm is brought to 95 degree elevation in flexion. For examining a right shoulder, the surgeon's left hand is placed behind the glenohumeral joint – that is, under the shoulder blade. The humeral head is then pushed posteriorly by holding the elbow with the surgeon's right hand and applying an axial load down the humerus, trying to push the humeral head backwards out of the joint. If the joint is posteriorly unstable, it will sublux at this stage and this may be detected by the examiner's left hand. However, it may not be picked up at this stage.

Keeping the compressive load applied down the shaft of the humerus, the latter is now brought around into a position of 90 degree abduction. If the shoulder was subluxed it will at this point relocate with a clunk just as in the 'load and shift' test. There is a real risk of producing a frank dislocation with the anterior and posterior stress tests, which does not matter in the anaesthetized patient, but is very embarrassing in the outpatient department, particularly if it can not be relocated!

Neurological assessment

Finally, the patient should have a rapid neurological assessment made of the rest of the arm, and the pulses and peripheral perfusion should be noted. If abnormal neurology is detected, for instance suprascapular nerve entrapment is suspected, then neurophysiological testing should be advised. Imaging is discussed in Chapter 3.

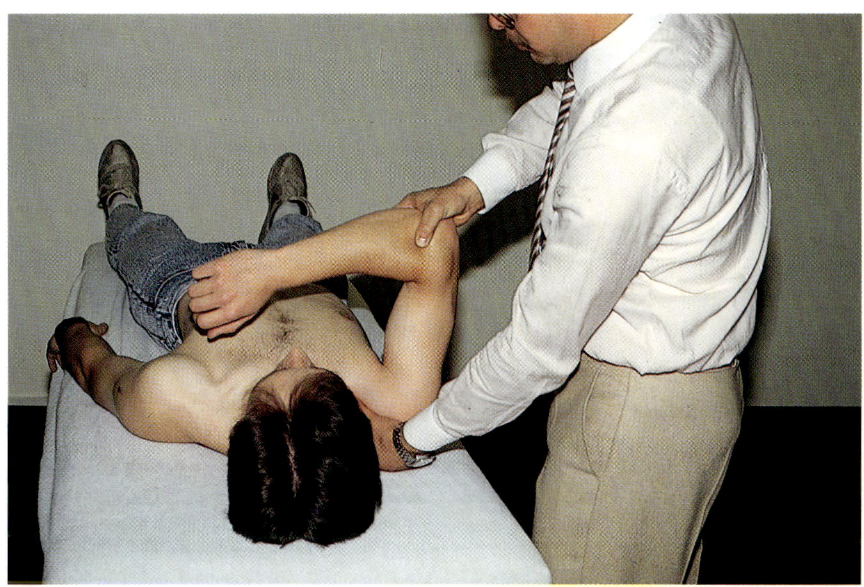

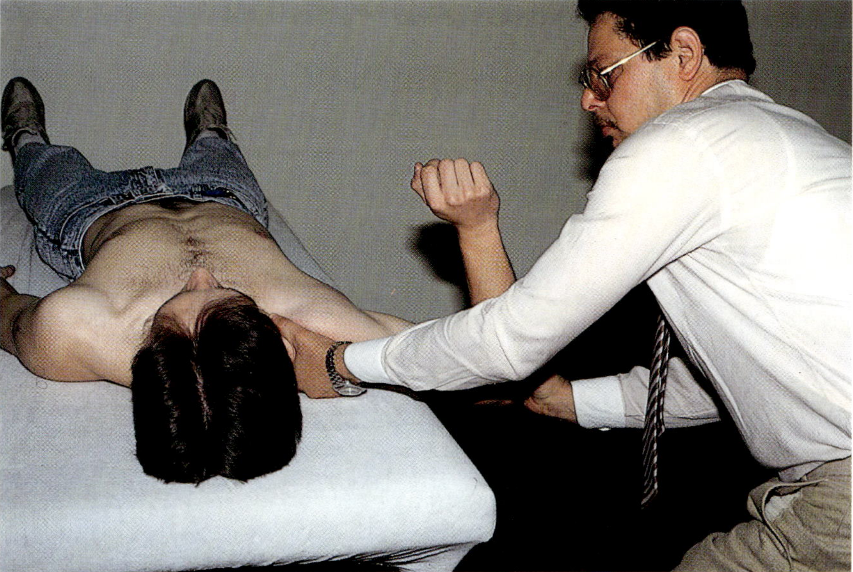

Figure 2.16a and b

Posterior stress test: with the patient lying supine the humerus is pushed out of the back into a subluxed position. Load is then applied to the joint and the humerus brought from 90 degrees of flexion to 90 degrees of abduction, which will reduce the subluxation with a palpable jerk.

3 Imaging the shoulder

Stephen Austin *MB BS, FRCR,*
Consultant Radiologist,
Great Ormond Street Hospital for Sick Children,
London

Introduction

For many years, plain X-rays were the only available means for imaging the shoulder and, as a result, there has been a tendency for radiologists to concentrate on bony aspects of shoulder joint pathology at the expense of the surrounding soft tissues. The newer imaging methods are much more sensitive to soft tissue abnormalities, and an impressive range of these techniques has been applied to shoulder imaging:

- plain radiography
- arthrography – single and double contrast
- CT arthrography
- digital subtraction arthrography
- subacromial bursography
- ultrasound
- magnetic resonance imaging (MRI)

Some of these methods (such as MRI) are still under evaluation, and others have found favour with a small number of enthusiasts (digital subtraction arthrography and subacromial bursography, for example). This chapter aims to review the available imaging modalities and to discuss the relative pros and cons of each technique.

Plain radiography

The standard anteroposterior (AP) and axial films of the shoulder will be the first imaging investigation for almost all patients presenting with shoulder disease. To get the most information out of these films, meticulous radiographic technique is essential.

The standard AP projection of the shoulder is taken with the patient slightly oblique, with the arm supinated, and in slight abduction, and should be centred to the coracoid process. The film should be exposed so as to demonstrate both bony and soft tissue detail (Figure 3.1). The acromion, and the greater and lesser tuberosities, should be visible. In the normal patient, the vertical distance between the inferior surface of the acromion, and the superior margin of the humeral head (the so-called acromiohumeral interval) should be at least 7 mm. A reduction in this measurement is suggestive of rotator cuff disease, although it is important to point out that this measurement can be artifactually reduced by radiographic factors, such as centring too low, for example. It is often possible to see a thin, dark line of fat in this region (the peribursal fat plane), which represents extrasynovial fat surrounding the

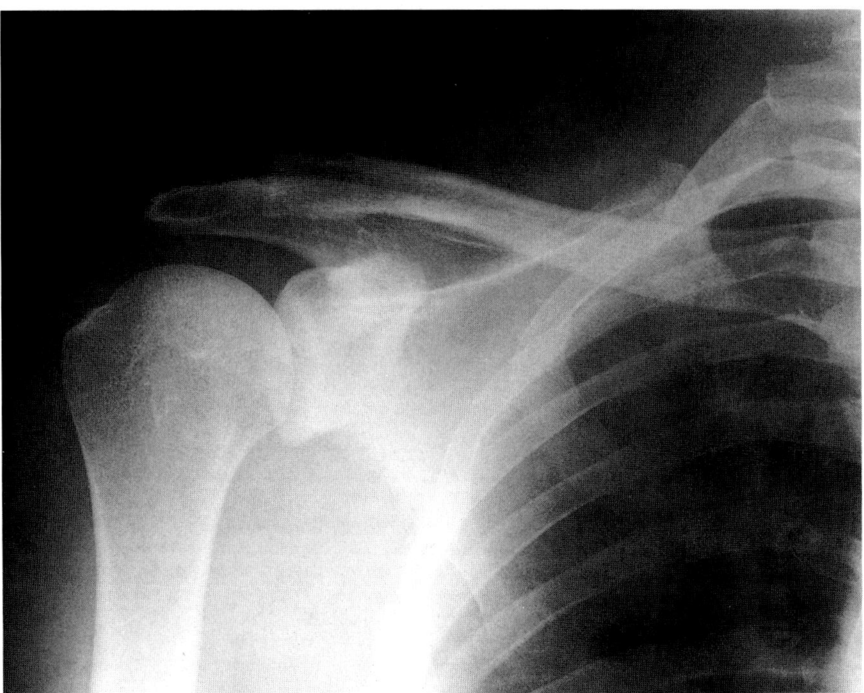

Figure 3.1
Standard AP radiograph of the shoulder.

subacromial/subdeltoid bursa. The fat line can be seen as a radiolucency lying deep to the deltoid and extending to the greater tuberosity. It is normally 1–2 mm thick, and is best seen in films taken in slight internal rotation. Failure to visualize the fat plane is a sensitive but non-specific sign of periarticular disease, including tears of the rotator cuff.[1]

The AP projection is of great value in the detection of soft tissue calcification (Figure 3.2). Many eponymous views have been described to assist in detecting hydroxyapatite deposition in different components of the rotator cuff. However, unless non-standard views are performed frequently, they are likely to be poorer in quality, and unfamiliar to their interpreters, which limits their value.

Figure 3.3 shows the standard axial view, which has been taken with the palm down. In this position, the greater tuberosity lies posteriorly, and the lesser anteriorly. In the injured patient, the standard axial view may be difficult to obtain. In these circumstances, a modified axial view, developed by Wallace and col-

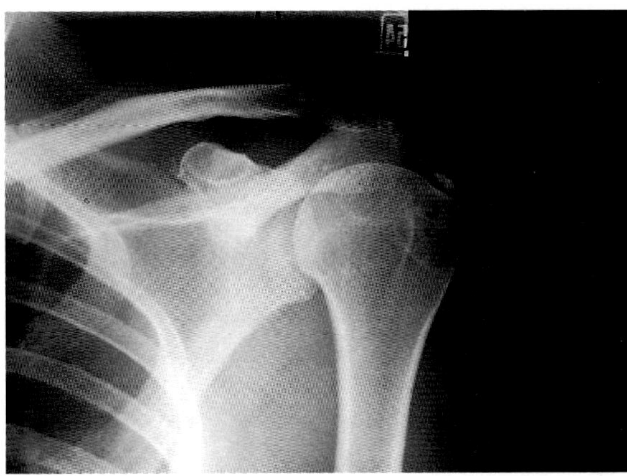

Figure 3.2

Soft tissue calcification on AP radiograph.

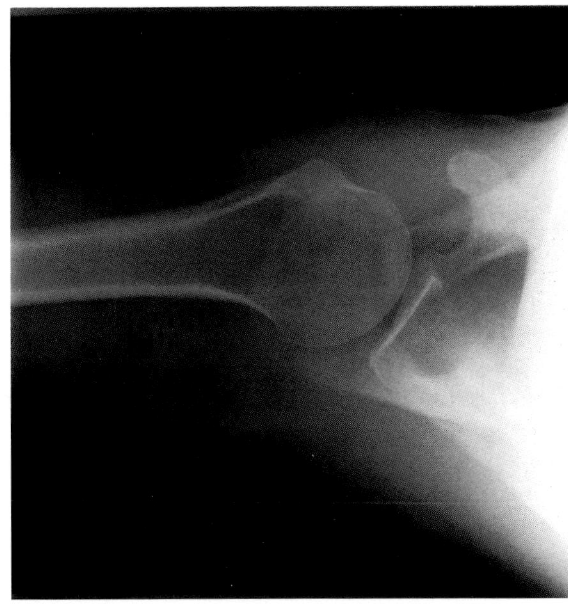

Figure 3.3

Standard axial view.

leagues [2] can be helpful. In this technique, the patient is sitting rotated, so that the scapula is parallel to the edge of the horizontal cassette, which is in contact with the arm. The tube is angled at 30 degrees. In this position, the central ray passes just lateral to the coracoid process, through the joint, to the cassette. The effect of this is to produce a magnified, and slightly distorted image of the shoulder (Figure 3.4), but with the advantage that the patient can be X-rayed without removing slings or collars and cuffs.

The search for the hatchet lesion, the humeral head defect produced by recurrent anterior dislocation, has generated a large number of eponymous radiographic projections. When the lesion is large, it can be demonstrated by an internally rotated AP projection, or a palm-down axial. More subtle lesions may require specialized techniques like the Stryker view, arthrography, or CT to demonstrate them.

A number of indirect plain film signs of rotator cuff disease have been described. In 1964, Cotton and Rideout[3] analysed over 100 cases, both radiologically and pathologically, at postmortem. They found that cyst formation in the upper two-thirds of the anatomical neck was a reliable and constant sign. The acromiohumeral interval was reduced in many cuff tears, but could be normal in the presence of severe disruption. Sclerosis of the greater tuberosity was a very unreliable sign, but sclerosis or remodelling of the inferior acromial surface correlated well with the presence of a cuff tear. The formation of a subacromial spur, an area of new bone formation arising from the inferior surface of the acromion[4] has also been described in some patients with full thickness tears.[5]

In general, plain films of the shoulder are of greatest value in acute trauma, and in the assessment of calcific periarthritis. Many abnormalities can be seen which suggest the presence of soft tissue disease, but these are usually non-specific, and the X-ray may be completely normal in the presence of a complete rotator cuff disruption.

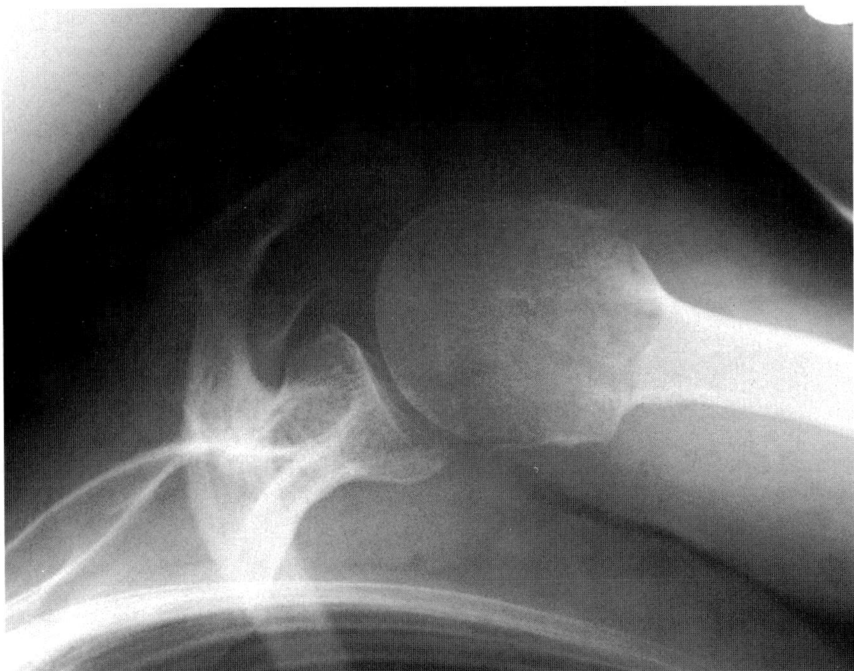

Figure 3.4
Nottingham axial view.

Arthrography

Arthrography is at present the most common special radiological investigation of the shoulder performed, and its practice is still on the increase, although there are suggestions that it may be supplanted by less invasive methods.[6] There are a number of different ways of performing a shoulder arthrogram. The single contrast technique, using iodinated contrast media alone, was first described in the 1930s,[7] but the double contrast technique (using less contrast, but with the addition of air) with erect filming provides better visualization of the soft tissue anatomy, and is now more widely performed.

Many different techniques for puncturing the joint are described, but the author uses an anterior approach,[8] which gives consistent results. After a standard series of control films, which include internal and external rotation AP films, and an axial film, the patient is placed supine on the X-ray screening table, with the arm elevated slightly, and in a neutral position. A point 2 cm lateral and below the coracoid is marked. The skin is cleaned and infiltrated with local anaesthetic, and a 21-gauge, short bevelled needle is advanced under screening control, with a slight medial inclination into the joint. A useful way of telling if the needle is in the joint is to fill the hub of the needle with local anaesthetic. When the capsule is punctured, the level of fluid will fall.

Five ml of positive contrast medium is then injected, followed by 15–20 ml of room air. If the needle is in the correct place, contrast will flow

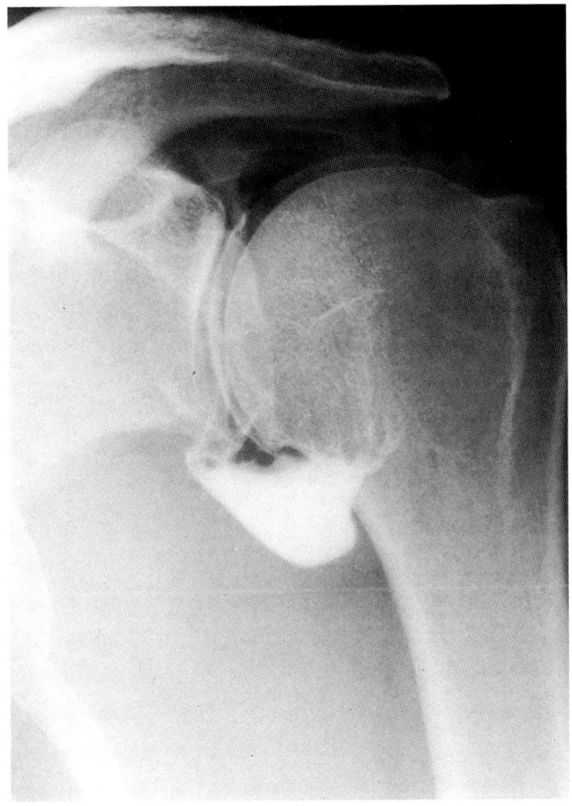

Figure 3.5

Normal shoulder arthrogram. Note that long head of biceps can be seen, as can the intra-articular triangle, into which the arthroscope is inserted.

into the axillary recess and subscapularis bursa. Gentle manipulation of the arm, and particularly adduction, may force contrast through a defect in the rotator cuff into the subacromial bursa, which does not normally fill. After contrast has been injected, a further series of films is taken, including erect films.

Figure 3.5 from a normal arthrogram series shows the contrast confined to the joint capsule, outlining the intra-articular portion of the tendon of the long head of biceps, and the tendon sheath. Contrast here outlines the deep surface of the rotator cuff, and there is no sign of contrast in the region of the subacromial bursa. Although non-filling of the tendon sheath was at one time regarded as abnormal, it is now known that this can be seen in up to 10 per cent of normal shoulders. Leakage of contrast from the biceps tendon sheath can also be seen occasionally, and this is also regarded as normal. In the presence of a full thickness cuff tear, the joint capsule is continuous with the subacromial or subdeltoid bursa, and contrast will enter this space.

On the internal rotation view (Figure 3.6) the superior surface of the cuff is demonstrated but is deficient at one point, which is the site of the defect. On internal rotation, the infraspinatus muscle is brought to lie laterally and under the acromion on the AP view, and if this does not appear intact, then the tear must be large in size. Sometimes, little contrast will enter the subacromial bursa, but the site and size of the tear will be well shown. Occasionally, with a small tear, positive contrast will not enter the subacromial bursa, but air will. This can easily be confused with the fat outlining the subdeltoid bursa, which is most easily seen on the internal rotation view. If there is any doubt, delayed films and/or CT should be performed.

Axial views with the double contrast method can demonstrate the glenoid labrum well, particularly the anterior portion, and this has been combined with conventional and computed tomography in the investigation of shoulder instability. Conventional arthrography has also been used in other clinical disorders, notably 'adhesive capsulitis', where a small-volume joint, with obliteration of normal synovial recesses, and lymphatic intravasation have been reported. This is one situation where the single contrast technique is probably superior. Treatment of the disorder by repeated capsular distension during arthrography has been described.[9]

The major disadvantages of arthrography for rotator cuff lesions are that partial thickness

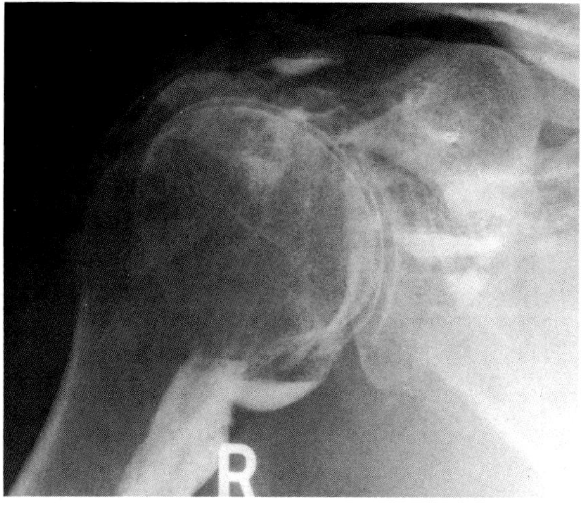

Figure 3.6
Arthrogram in internal rotation showing rotator cuff tear, with leak of contrast material into the subacromial bursa. Contrast has also leaked down the biceps tunnel (which is normal) and then escaped.

Figure 3.7
Normal CT arthrogram of the shoulder showing anterior and posterior aspects of the labrum.

tears will only be shown if they involve the deep surface of the cuff, and these only occasionally. Partial tears involving the superficial surface or body of the cuff cannot be demonstrated. In addition, filling of the subacromial bursa is not unusual following a successful rotator cuff repair, so that the technique is not as helpful in the assessment of postoperative problems. However, it is quick and simple to perform, requires little or no specialized equipment, and has a very low complication rate.

CT arthrography

The arthrographic technique is slightly modified if CT is used, with typically only 1–2 ml of positive contrast and 10–15 ml of air being injected. Thin slices (3–5 mm) are obtained through the shoulder joint, with the arm in slight internal rotation. Selected slices may be repeated with the arm in external rotation to demonstrate the posterior labrum more effectively.[10] This normal example (Figure 3.7) shows both the anterior and posterior aspects of the labrum.

The main use of the technique is in the investigation of recurrent shoulder instability. Hatchet deformities of the humeral head are well demonstrated by this method. All lesions were detected by CT arthrography, and there were no false positives in those patients in whom surgical confirmation was available in the above quoted series.

Bony glenoid rim (Bankart) lesions are also clearly seen, but one of the major advantages of the technique is the ability to demonstrate abnormalities of the glenoid labrum. Compared with surgery or arthroscopy, the sensitivity for detection of labral detachment or tears using the technique is close to 100 per cent, particularly for the anterior portion. Humeral head lesions are exceptionally well demonstrated by this technique, as are abnormalities of the biceps tendon.

Digital subtraction arthrography

This method uses digital subtraction techniques taken from the field of angiography, and requires expensive specialized equipment. It involves injection of contrast into the joint, while keeping the arm still, and taking images at 1 second intervals. The images are then subtracted by a computer from a mask image without contrast, in order to obtain bone-free images. Enthusiasts claim that it is more sensitive in detecting full thickness and deep surface tears, and can show the site and size of a tear more accurately than the conventional technique. It can also be used to evaluate shoulder replacements for loosening. It is technically more difficult than conventional arthrography, and has not found wide application.

Subacromial bursography

The subacromial bursa may be entered inadvertently during conventional arthrography, but direct injection has been used to demonstrate cuff tears, and particularly those partial tears of the superficial surface of the cuff which cannot be shown by conventional arthrography. It has also been used in the investigation of impingement syndrome, when pooling of contrast in the subdeltoid part of the subacromial bursa during abduction and external rotation is noted.[5] The technique is rather more difficult than shoulder arthrography, and the normal bursa can be problematic to find with a needle. It is not widely practised, and many reports of its use come from Japan, where it has also been used in the diagnosis of adhesive capsulitis.

Ultrasound

Ultrasound is not a technique commonly associated with orthopaedics, although interest in the technique is growing. Ultrasound of the rotator cuff was first described in 1984.[11] However, the advance of technology has been such that the development of high resolution scanners and high frequency probes, typically 7.5–10 MHz, has improved the accuracy of the technique. The advantages of the technique are that it is quick and non-invasive, and it is easy to examine both shoulders at one sitting. Images can be obtained in several different planes.

The technique has the potential to demonstrate partial thickness tears. Figure 3.8 is an example of a normal cuff in the coronal plane, with the greater tuberosity, and the deltoid muscle lying superficially. Images are also obtained in the sagittal plane, and transversely. It is also important to observe the cuff during rotation of the shoulder. The criteria used to diagnose a cuff tear are controversial. There is general agreement that visualization of a defect, or non-visualization of the cuff as in Figure 3.9 where only the deltoid is visible, and no cuff can be seen, are reliable criteria for the diagnosis of a cuff tear.

The significance of areas of altered echogenicity (Figure 3.10) is less certain. Some may represent full thickness and some partial thickness tears, but the changes are not consistent, and alterations in echogenicity alone should not

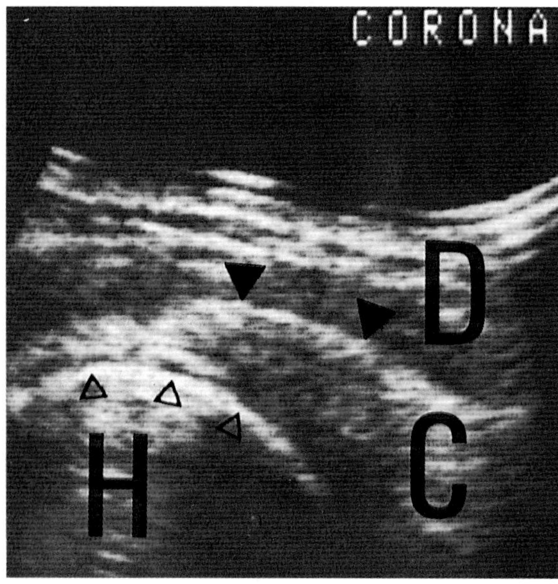

Figure 3.8

Normal rotator cuff on coronal ultrasound: right shoulder seen from in front. D = Deltoid, C = Rotator cuff, H = Humeral head.

be used as the sole criterion for diagnosis.[12] Areas of fibrosis or calcification can also produce abnormal echogenic areas.[13] In one prospective series of 51 shoulders, ultrasound had a sensitivity of 100 per cent for the detection of a cuff tear, but the specificity was only 75 per cent, and the overall accuracy 92 per cent. The major disadvantages of the technique are the time it takes to learn the method, and the fact that arthrography may still be required before surgery. It is sufficiently sensitive to exclude serious cuff tears with confidence in good hands.

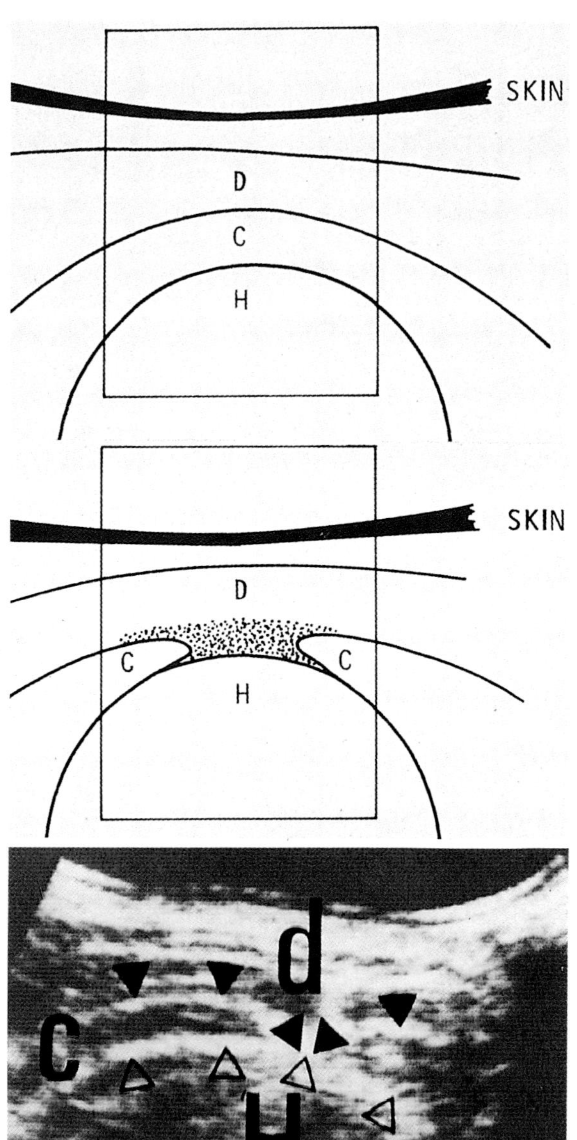

Figure 3.9

Full thickness rotator cuff tear on sonography (sagittal scan). Top shows line diagram of the normal normal appearance. Middle shows line diagram of rotator cuff tear. Bottom shows sonogram of rotator cuff tear (dark arrows top of cuff and tear, light arrows bottom of cuff). D = Deltoid, C = Cuff, H = Humeral head.

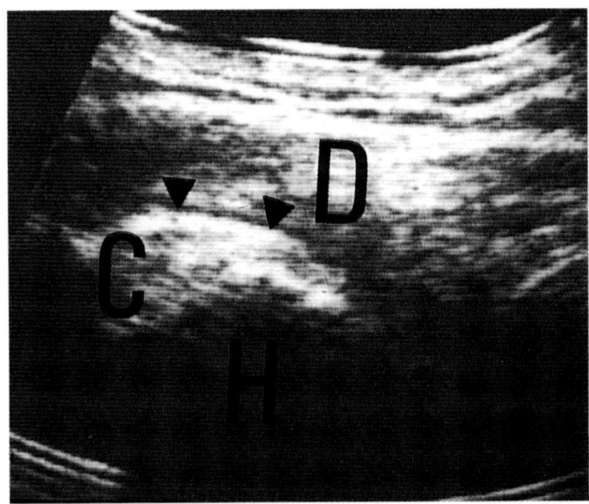

Figure 3.10
Coronal scan of left shoulder showing a highly echoic insertion of the supraspinatus tendon.

There have been reports of the use of ultrasound in the evaluation of the postoperative shoulder. This is a situation in which arthrography is less helpful, as a successfully repaired cuff may still leak contrast. Unfortunately, postoperative changes in cuff echogenicity are common, and acromioplasty removes a normal ultrasonic landmark, making it difficult to separate cuff from overlying deltoid. Nevertheless, if the criteria of non-visualization, or demonstration of a defect are used, the technique is highly accurate in the diagnosis of recurrent tears.[14]

Magnetic resonance imaging (MRI)

With the development of high field NMR scanners and improved surface coil technology, it has become feasible over the last few years to undertake high resolution shoulder MRI. The peripheral location, and unique anatomy of the shoulder joint does pose some technical problems for MRI, however. Surface coils are essential to provide high spatial resolution, and novel coils have been designed specifically for shoulder imaging.[15] Software modifications may also be required (for example, to alter the centre frequency) to allow off-centre zooming.[16] T_2-weighted images are essential, but either T_1-weighted or proton density images are also important to assess morphology, and the subdeltoid fat plane. Axial images are obtained, as well as coronal oblique images, in the plane of the supraspinatus tendon, and sagittal oblique images, perpendicular to this plane (Figure 3.11).

Like ultrasound, there is no clear consensus on the criteria for diagnosis of a tear. T_2-weighted spin echo images frequently show areas of high signal within the cuff, but some of these patients will prove to have intact cuffs at surgery. In general, a normal intensity cuff with a normal subdeltoid fat plane is likely to be normal. An area of increased signal in the region of the cuff on T_2-weighted images, with normal morphology, and a normal subdeltoid fat plane probably indicates cuff degeneration without a tear. Most patients with a cuff tear show increased cuff signal, or discontinuity. Loss of the subdeltoid fat plane or fluid in the subacromial bursa on T_2-weighted images are also very suggestive findings.[17]

In most of the published series, MRI compares favourably with arthrography, although there are always a few tears missed by MRI, but shown by arthrography.[18] Some partial thickness tears are only demonstrated by MRI, however. In impingement syndrome, MRI

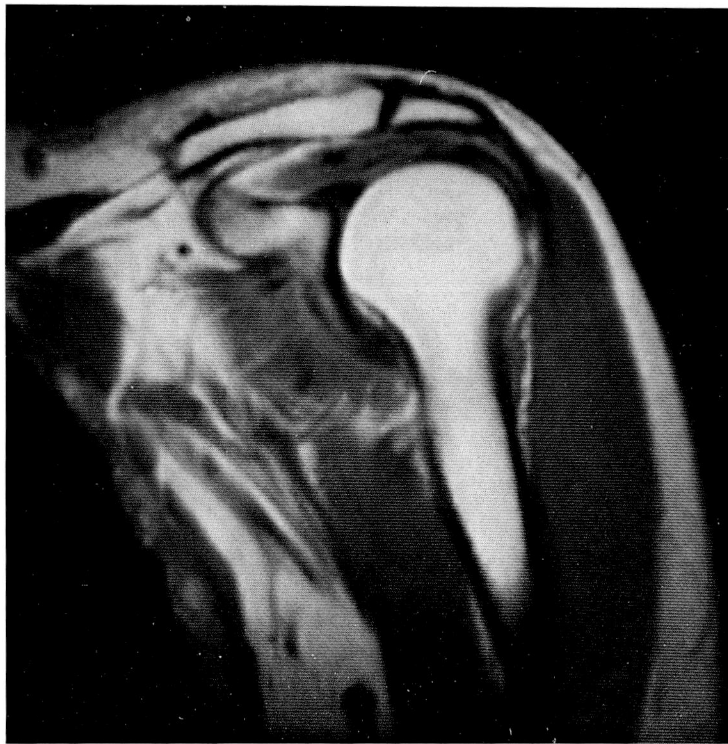

Figure 3.11
Coronal T_1-weighted spin-echo image of a normal shoulder showing the long head of biceps, and the rotator cuff lying between the joint and the subdeltoid bursa.

proved very sensitive to cuff degeneration in one series.[19] However, subacromial injection of steroids can produce MRI changes which mimic cuff pathology. This is a potential drawback, as many patients will have had local injections before being referred for MRI.

Results in recurrent shoulder dislocation are less encouraging, as the normal glenoid labrum is a low intensity structure on most sequences, and is consequently harder to assess. CT arthrography may be more sensitive in the detection of labral pathology, although it can be demonstrated by MRI. Similar reservations also apply to the diagnosis of capsular stripping on MRI. This is readily demonstrated by CT arthrography, as the joint is distended during the procedure. MRI can only detect capsular separation in the presence of a joint effusion.[20] The accuracy of MRI in the detection of humeral head defects is probably equal to that of CT arthrography.

Conclusion

Imaging techniques based on X-rays are still the mainstay of shoulder investigation. Newer methods such as ultrasound and MRI have certain limitations, but have much to offer in terms of soft tissue detail, and are continually improving, as well as providing information unavailable by other methods.

4 Clinical procedure

Theatre organization

Arthroscopic surgery of the shoulder is a highly technical and demanding form of surgery. It requires special instrumentation and a highly skilled team consisting of surgeon, anaesthetist, scrub nurse and circulating nurse. Diagnostic arthroscopy of the shoulder, on the other hand, requires little more than an arthroscope, light source and hook probe, as well as a large helping of enthusiasm and determination on the part of the surgeon, and tolerance from the anaesthetist and the nursing team. Initially even diagnostic arthroscopy takes time, and the goodwill of the operating team is increased if they can all follow events on a television monitor.

Since shoulder arthroscopy is a very specialized form of surgery, it is best performed in a dedicated day-case arthroscopy suite. Failing this, a good-sized general or orthopaedic theatre, with nurses trained in arthroscopic techniques of the knee, is the next best situation. To perform this type of surgery in a general surgical theatre with untrained staff needs an extremely optimistic outlook from the surgeon!

The surgeon should have a good training in arthroscopic surgery of the knee before undertaking arthroscopy of the shoulder, and this must be combined with an extensive knowledge of shoulder anatomy, pathology, and an ability to undertake open surgery of the shoulder in an experienced and competent fashion. The surgeon should then attend a shoulder arthroscopy course, and practise on shoulder models before attempting any form of arthroscopic procedure on the shoulder of a patient. The surgeon may wish to practise on cadaver shoulders but, unless very fresh cadavers are used, the shoulder soon shrinks and becomes difficult to move, and the whole process becomes rather sordid. It is far better to practise on models and to gain experience by assisting a surgeon who is competent in this technique.

A good theatre layout is shown in Figure 4.1 and is based on the dedicated suite of Dr L. Johnson's unit, at Ingham Medical Center, Lansing, Michigan. The patient lies in the lateral decubitus position with the surgeon directly behind his/her shoulder. A Mayo stand with the principal arthroscopic equipment required for the procedure is placed directly opposite the surgeon, and the scrub nurse stands alongside the Mayo stand ready to hand instruments to the surgeon when needed. Directly beyond the instruments is the television stand on which are placed the television monitor, camera equipment, light source, shaver system and video recorder. The arm of the patient is supported by a shoulder holder. An extra Mayo stand with

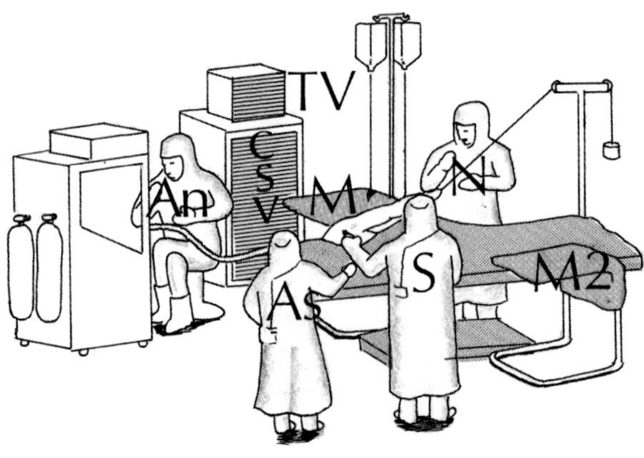

Figure 4.1

Suggested theatre setup for shoulder arthroscopy. An, Anaesthetist; N, Nurse; S, Surgeon; A, Assistant; M and M2, Mayo stands; TV, Television monitor; CSV, Camera, Shaver, Video.

accessory instruments is placed to the right of the surgeon and the first assistant stands to the surgeon's left.

Equipment

For diagnostic shoulder arthroscopy

A standard 30 degree knee arthroscope is used for shoulder arthroscopy. The shoulder is a large joint and we have found that a small diameter arthroscope gives too small a picture of the joint, as well as having difficulty delivering enough light to illuminate the far recesses of the joint cavity. Obviously a good light source and either sterile saline or Hartmann's solution is required along with the arthroscope. The only other piece of equipment needed is a wide-bore needle to establish an outflow, and a hook probe.

For arthroscopic surgery of the shoulder

Basics

For simple surgery, such as the removal of loose bodies and synovial biopsies, the only equipment needed are the standard arthroscopic tools of the trade as used for knee surgery, in particular a pair of arthroscopic grasping forceps, basket forceps and small pituitary rongeurs (Figure 4.2).

Television system

For any form of more complex surgery, a television system is mandatory. Again any system that works for the knee will work for the shoulder. There have been rapid advances in camera technology recently and, in buying a camera system, the minimal requirements are a lightweight balanced camera head capable of repeated immersion for sterilization, with a white set memory to establish colour balance, allied to a high intensity light source and high resolution colour monitor.

If the shoulder is being arthroscoped in the normal lateral position, then the television monitor should be placed opposite the surgeon, the centre of the screen being on a level with the surgeon's eye. One problem that arises in shoulder arthroscopy is that if the arthroscope is changed from the routine posterior portal to the anterior portal, the surgeon can feel awkward still looking forward at the monitor in front of him. Body image becomes distorted and triangulation difficult, similar to attempting to perform internal fixation of a femoral neck fracture under image intensifier control with the intensifier image upside down and back to front. The dedicated arthroscopist will have a second monitor stationed behind him and, when he changes to the anterior portal, he then looks over his shoulder at the second monitor, or moves to the other side of the operating table

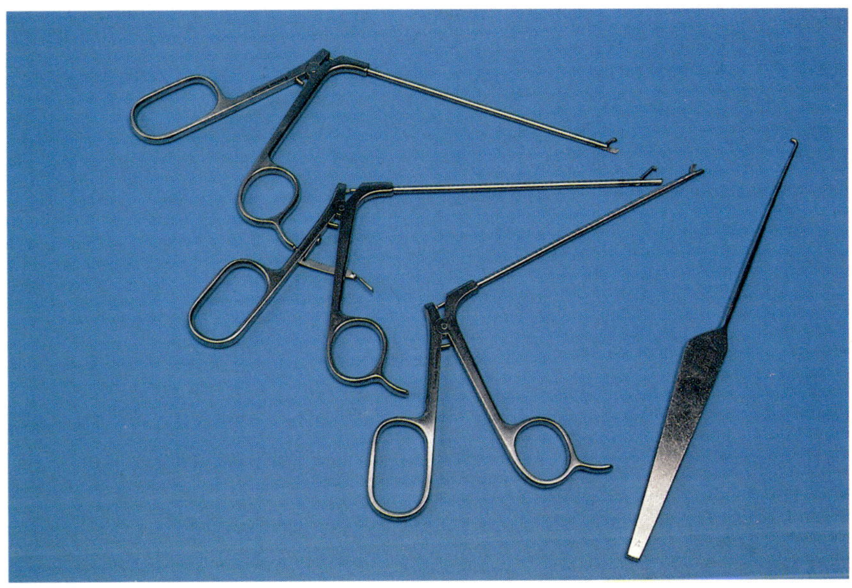

Figure 4.2
Basic instruments: from left, scissors, graspers, basket forceps, and hook probe.

and looks at the second monitor, in order to overcome 'body image' problems.

Once a good television system has been purchased, it costs little more to link a video recorder into the system to get a permanent record of the procedures. For the surgeon who has everything, this system can be linked to printers and recorders which can store images on computer disk, or reproduce them as slides, prints, transparencies, or videotape recordings. A character generator can also be used to identify each recording.

Whereas a large amount of arthroscopic surgery of the knee can be performed with hand-operated instruments, arthroscopic surgery of the shoulder really requires powered instrumentation. Powered systems mean that there is less need for instruments to be passed in and out of the joint, for, with most of these systems, the excised tissue is sucked out of the joint down the shaver or bur shaft. This is important, as the shoulder is surrounded by a greater mass of soft tissue than the knee, making entry more difficult and more traumatic to the tissues. The fewer times a portal is transgressed, the better for the shoulder.

Arthroscopic subacromial decompression can be performed with a powered soft tissue resector and powered burs alone (see Chapter 8). However, the amount of bleeding, and therefore the time taken to complete the procedure, is reduced if an electrosurgical apparatus is used to define the area of resection and cut the soft tissue off the undersurface of the acromion first (Figure 4.3).

Shoulder repair is dependent upon very specialized equipment, and the choice depends upon the surgeon's philosophy regarding method of repair (see Chapter 7). For staple repair, Instrument Makar staples are needed (Figure 4.4); for the Caspari-type repair, the Caspari punch is needed (Figure 4.5) and, for the Morgan suture technique, Bowen needles are required (Figure 4.6). Many new techniques are being developed and there is no doubt that these will require specialized instruments of their own.

Arthroscopic photography

Good documentation of shoulder arthroscopy still requires 35 mm photography, although computer technology may soon make this redundant and allow high quality hard copy to be made from videotapes. It is really essential to have a power winder, or two hands will have to be used on the camera body and contamination of the arthroscope may occur as the surgeon's natural reaction is to steady the arthroscope itself for the next shot. High-speed film is needed, such as 1000 or 640 ASA tungsten film.

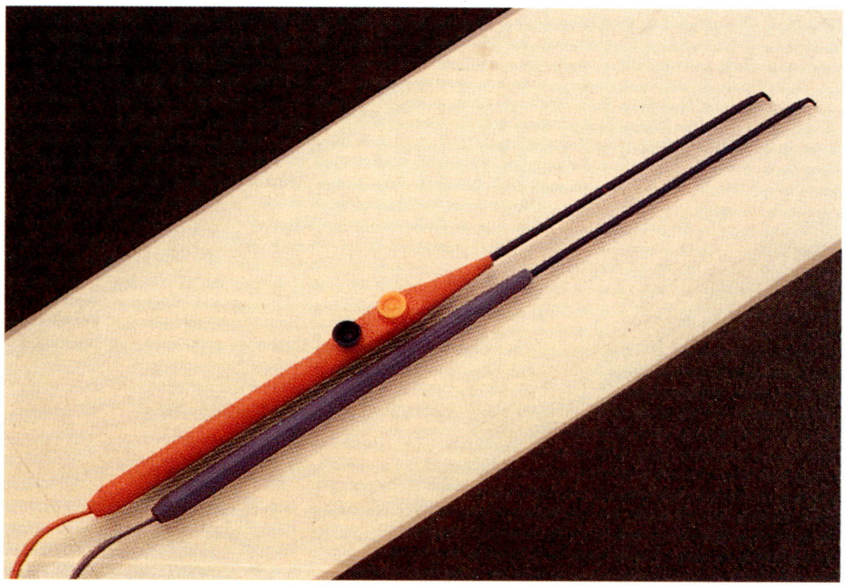

Figure 4.3
Electrosurgical apparatus is useful for subacromial decompression.

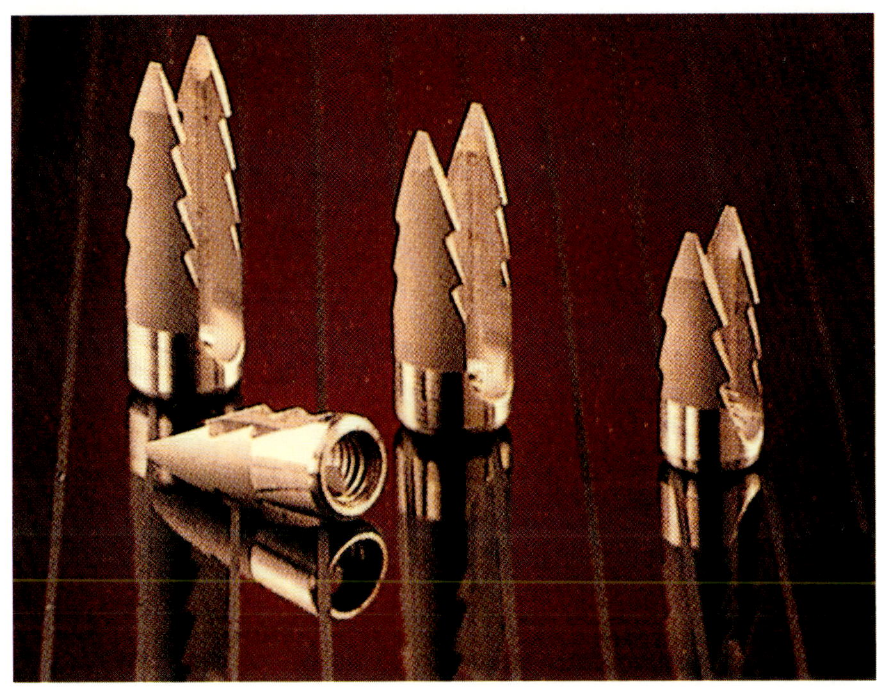

Figure 4.4
The Instrument Makar arthroscopic staple.

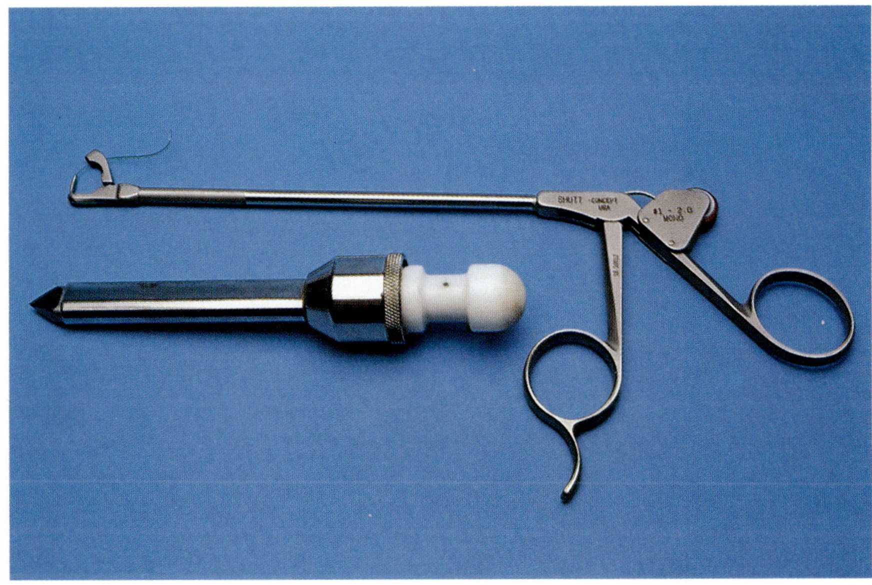

Figure 4.5
The Caspari suture punch for suture repair.

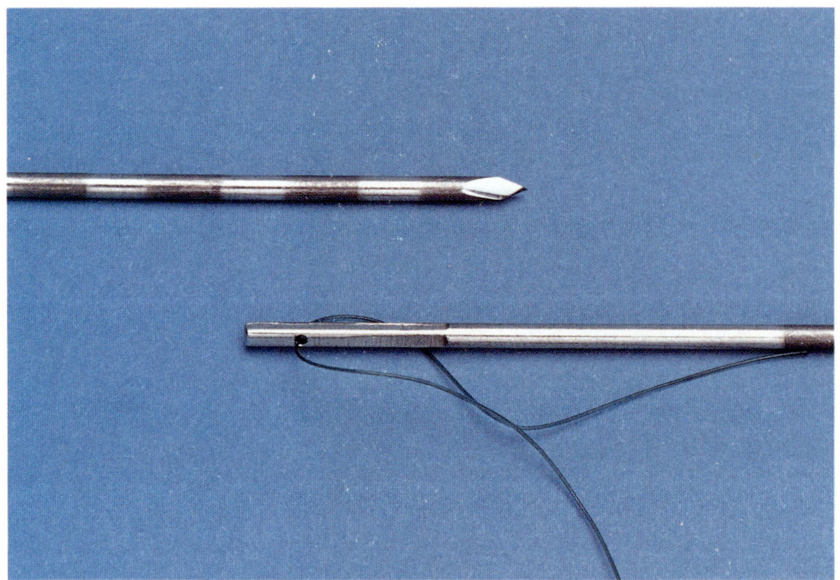

Figure 4.6
Bowen needles for suture repair.

Shoulder holders

A shoulder holder is a suspension device for the arm, used to distract the glenohumeral joint. They vary from the homemade bent piece of tubing (Figure 4.7) to extremely sophisticated devices such as the electrically switched and vacuum-powered arthrobot (Figure 4.8).

Great concern has been expressed about the relationship between postoperative nerve palsies and the use and duration of pull from shoulder holders during shoulder arthroscopy. Paulos et al[1] reported a 30 per cent incidence of transient paraesthesias following shoulder arthroscopy and Andrews, Carson and Ortega[2] implicated traction as a cause of ulnar and musculocutaneous neuropraxias during shoulder arthroscopies.

Klein, France and Mutschler[3] performed a series of experiments to measure the strain on the brachial plexus exerted by a shoulder holder. They mounted strain gauges to the upper trunk, lateral cord, median nerve and radial nerve of five fresh cadavers, which were then put in the lateral decubitus position for shoulder arthroscopy and the strain on the plexus measured in relation to arm position and load. They concluded that the best position of the arm in terms of maximum visibility associated with minimum strain on the plexus was

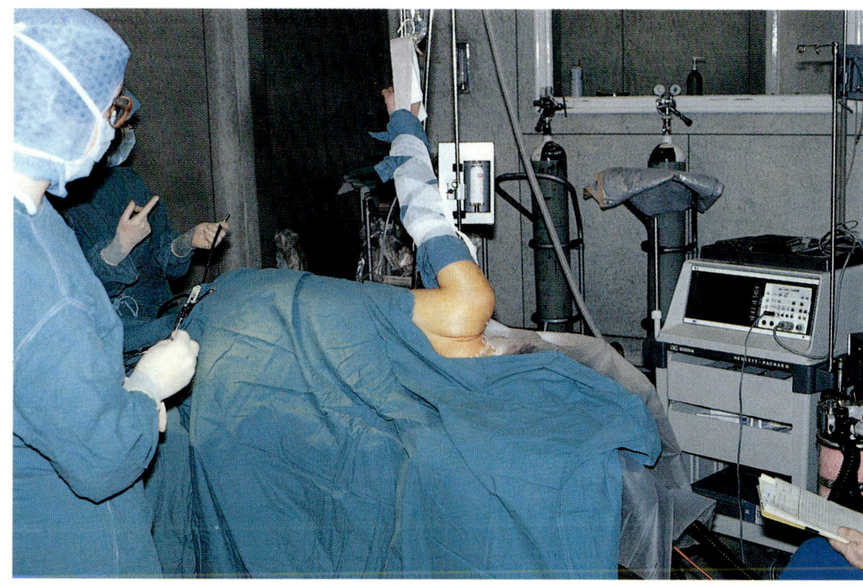

Figure 4.7

A very crude shoulder holder can be made from a bent pipe or a drip stand.

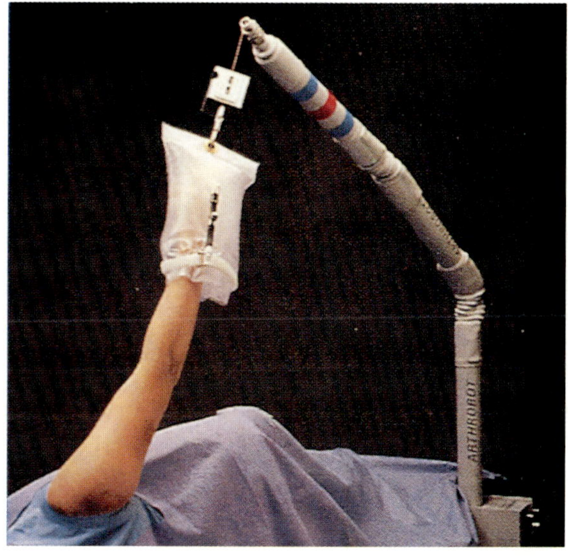

Figure 4.8

The arthrobot is a highly sophisticated shoulder holder.

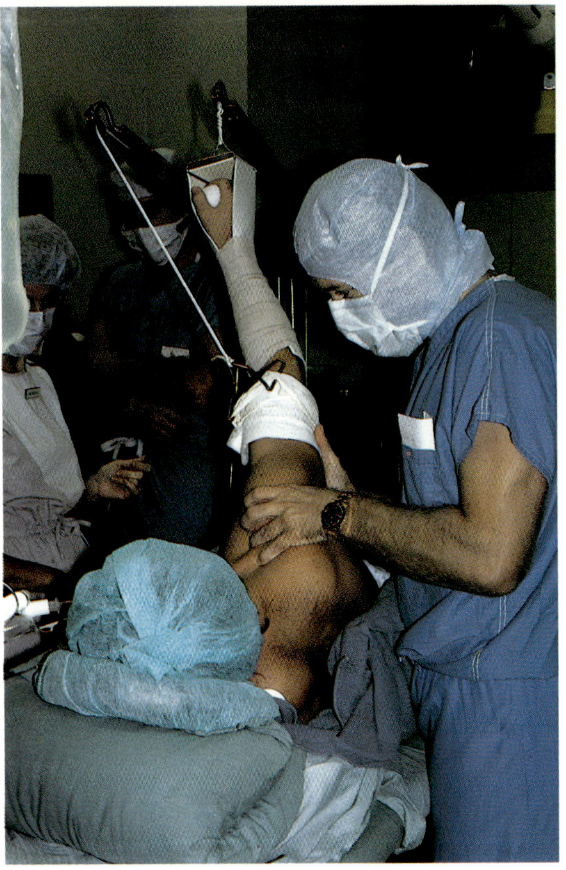

Figure 4.9

Two shoulder holders can be used to reduce pressure on the brachial plexus and distract the glenohumeral joint more thoroughly.

either 45 degrees of forward flexion and 90 degrees of abduction, or 45 degrees of forward flexion and 0 degrees of abduction.

Andrews et al[2] suggest that the best position for the arm is at 60–70 degrees of abduction and 15 degrees of forward flexion with 4.5–9 kg weight applied to the traction apparatus. Caspari[4] also feels that a traction apparatus is essential because traction supplied by an assistant is inconsistent and wanes as the assistant tires. Matthews[5] suggests that the arm should be placed in 45–60 degrees of abduction and 15 degrees of flexion, but that no more than 4.5 kg weight should be used. Matthews[6] has also shown how abduction should be released before proceeding to subacromial endoscopy as, with the arm at the side, the volume of the subacromial space is doubled from the volume with the arm at 45 degrees of abduction. For arthroscopic repair of the shoulder, Matthews uses not one but two shoulder holders (Figure 4.9), the second distracting the glenohumeral joint and being attached to the arm at the mid-humeral level. It is essential, if using a two-holder technique, to pad the humerus copiously in order to prevent neuropraxia to the median and ulnar nerves.

Gross and Fitzgibbons[7] also recommend applying the traction perpendicular to the humerus rather than along the line of the arm. They suggest that this elevates the humerus from the glenoid rather than distracting it into a subluxed position. This accentuates labral pathology and allows for better visualization of the lower third of the glenoid rim, while causing very little strain on the brachial plexus. They suggest that this should eliminate traction neuropraxias.

Preoperative procedures

Anaesthesia

Local anaesthesia may be used for shoulder arthroscopy and Warren et al[8] have reported a series of 44 arthroscopic subacromial decompressions performed under scalene block without anaesthetic problems. However, general anaesthesia for shoulder arthroscopy is preferable. General anaesthesia prevents embarrassment to the surgeon and loss of faith by the patient during the learning curve of the procedure, when the surgeon's dexterity may not match the patient's expectations! It is essential that the patient is intubated in order to remove both the anaesthetist and the anaesthetic equipment from the operative field, and to allow the surgeon to reach across the patient's head. The patient should be adequately monitored and all pressure areas should be properly padded.

When the lateral decubitus position is used, an axillary roll should be placed under the patient in order to prevent undue strain being placed on the brachial plexus of the unoperated side (Figure 4.10).

Positioning

The usual position for shoulder arthroscopy is the lateral decubitus position. A pillow is placed between the legs to prevent undue pressure and the trunk is supported with well-padded surgical posts (see Figure 4.10). If diagnostic arthroscopy alone is being undertaken, there is no need for a shoulder holder to be used, as the surgical assistant can provide distraction when needed. However, if arthroscopic surgery of the shoulder is being undertaken, then the arm should be connected to the shoulder holder using a proprietary traction apparatus.

Skyhar et al[9] have described the use of a 'beach-chair' or sitting position for shoulder arthroscopy. They have used this position for over 50 consecutive patients for arthroscopic

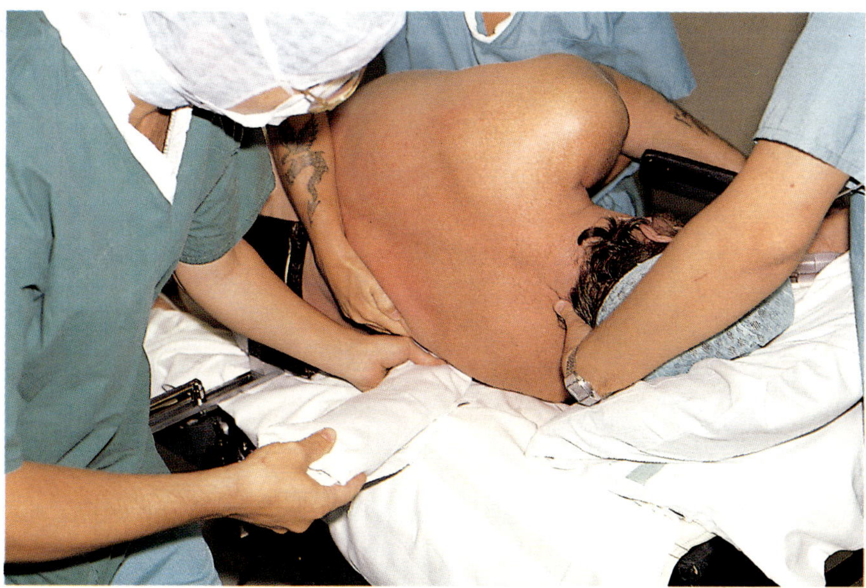

Figure 4.10

An axillary roll is placed under the patient to protect the brachial plexus of the unoperated side.

debridement, arthroscopic subacromial decompressions and arthroscopic shoulder stabilizations. Matthews[6] also suggests that a 'beach-chair' position be used for subacromial decompression as this increases the subacromial space and allows easier access if the shoulder or subacromial space requires open surgery. Gross and Fitzgibbons[7] suggest that the lateral decubitus position should be modified to a semilateral position by letting the patient rotate 30–40 degrees posteriorly. This places the glenoid parallel to the floor, which allows more comfortable arthroscopy and instrumentation.

Even with the use of television apparatus, arthroscopic techniques are not always as aseptic as open orthopaedic procedures. Therefore, if there is a need to proceed to open surgery, it is better to treat the open procedure as an entirely new operation. The patient should be repositioned, reprepared and draped, all instruments should be changed and the surgeon will need to rescrub and gown.

Draping the patient

The whole of the shoulder, arm and hand of the side to be arthroscoped is prepared with chlorhexidine in spirit, paying particular attention to the axilla. The preparation must extend to the midline of the chest to back and front, and include the neck (see Figure 4.11). A glove is placed over the hand, after preparation, and the arm is held by the assistant. A stockinette is then rolled down the arm (Figure 4.12).

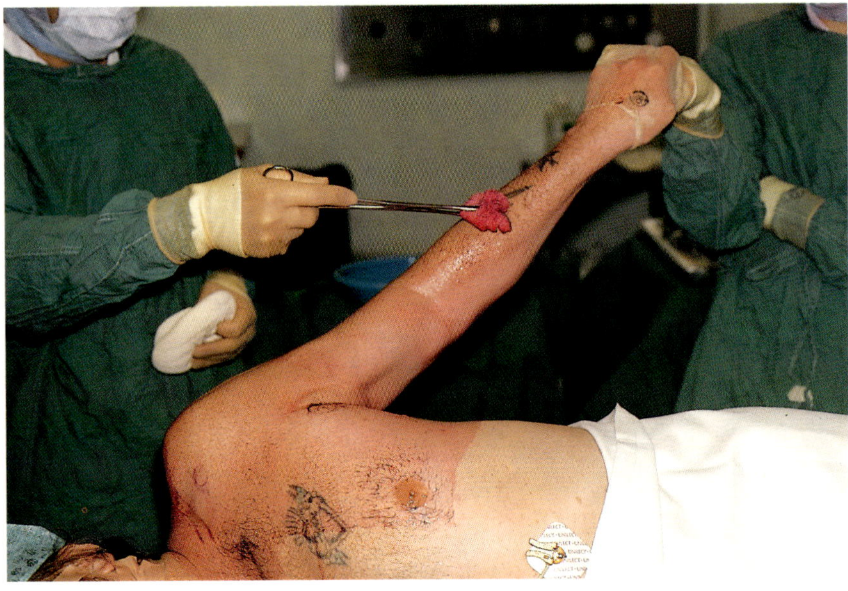

Figure 4.11

Preparation of the skin must be adequate, extending to the midline and up onto the neck.

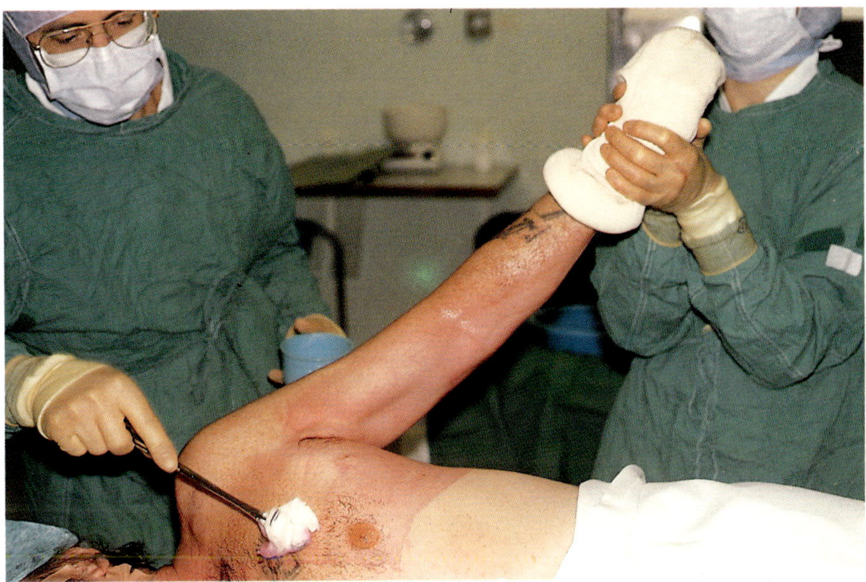

Figure 4.12
After the hand has been prepared, a stockinette is rolled down the arm.

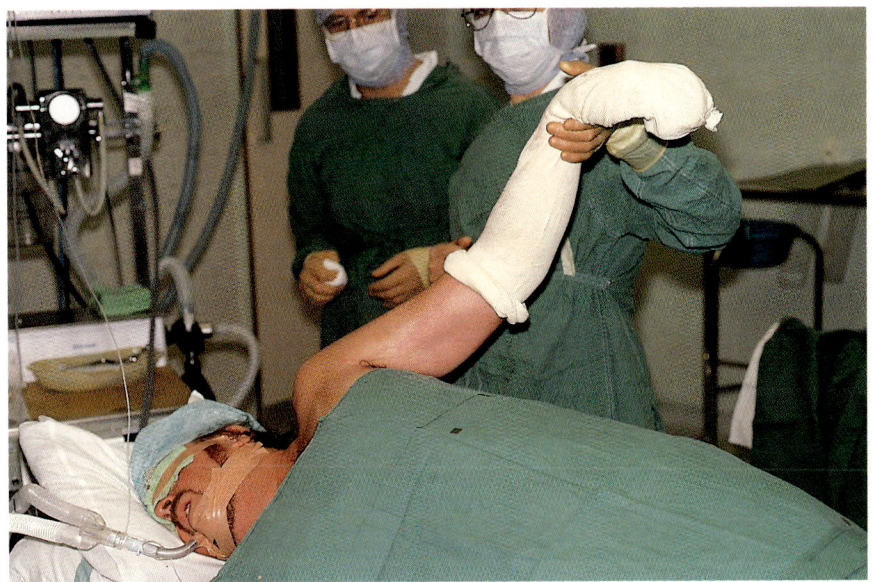

Figure 4.13
Drapes are then placed over the patient's body, from the axilla down.

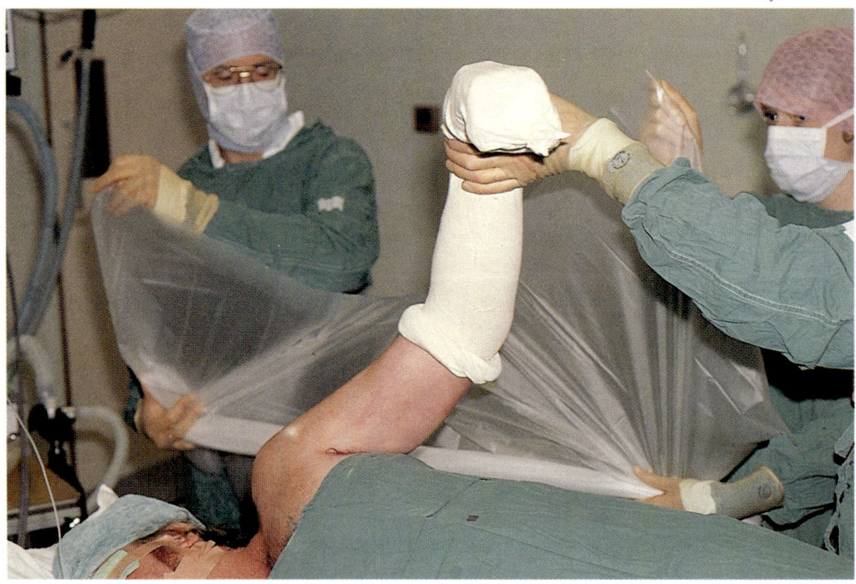

Figure 4.14

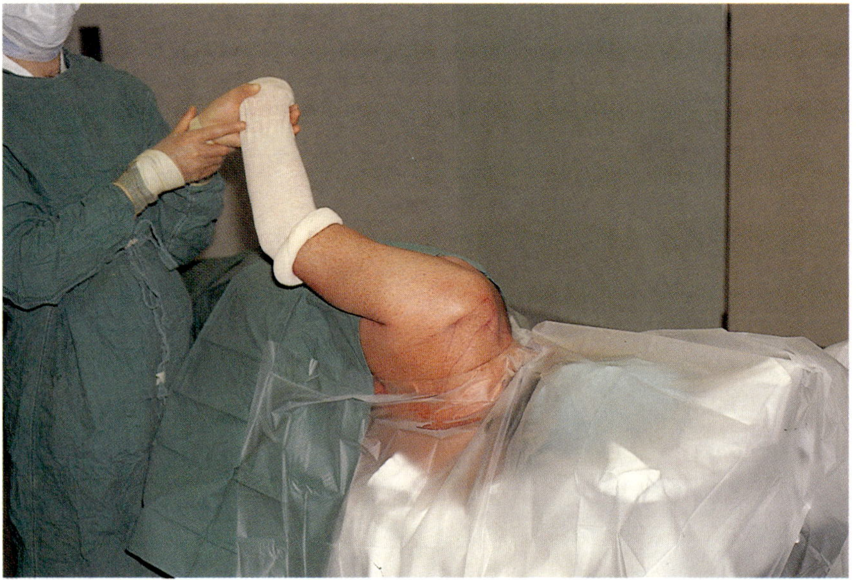

Figures 4.14 and 4.15

A sterile 'U-drape' is placed to prevent irrigation fluid leaking over the patient's hair and face during the procedure.

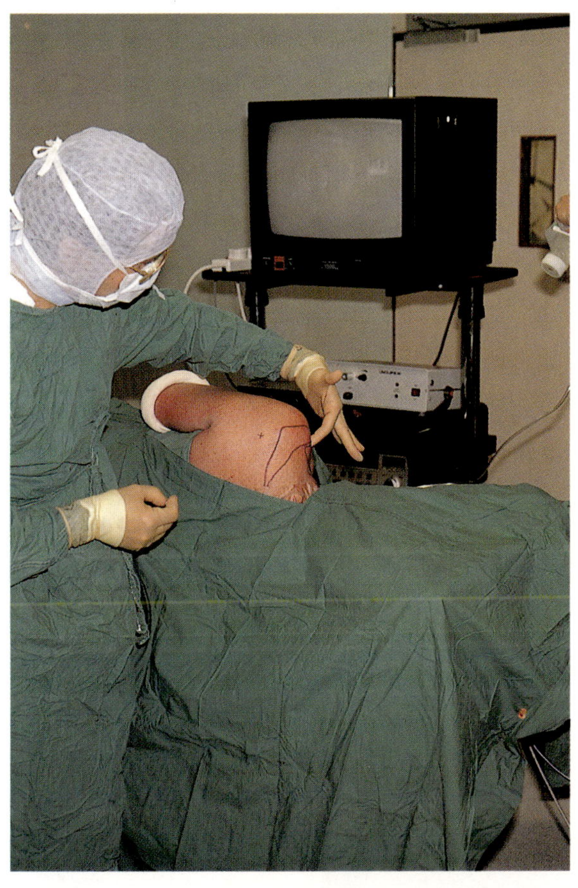

Figure 4.16

Draping is completed with an arm drape through which the arm is placed.

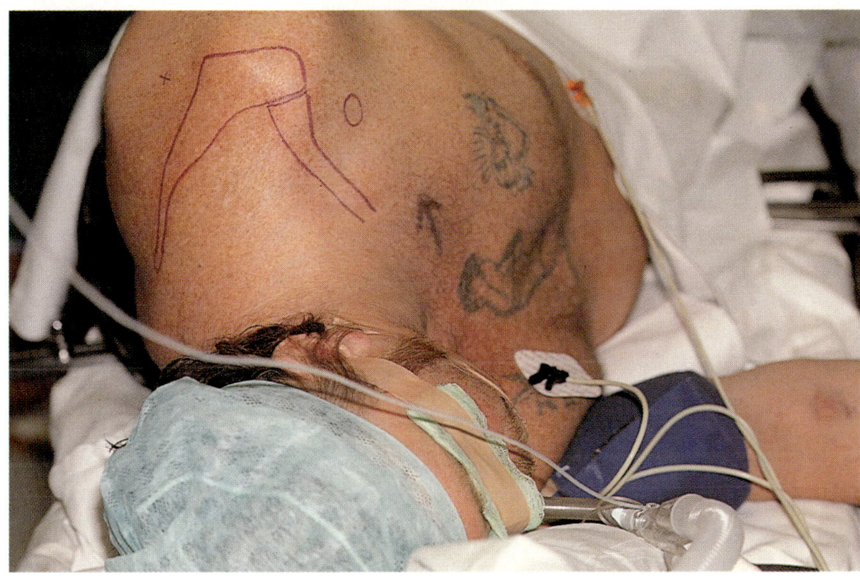

Figure 4.17

When starting to perform shoulder arthroscopies, it is useful to mark the landmarks of the acromion, the clavicle and the coracoid with a skin marking pen prior to portal placement.

The draping starts with waterproof drapes being placed to cover the patient's body, from the axilla downwards (Figure 4.13). A waterproof 'U-drape' is then placed over the patient's head to prevent irrigation fluid and blood from reaching the unprepared parts of the patient (Figures 4.14 and 4.15). A further drape with a hole in the centre is then placed over the arm (Figure 4.16). The skin markings of the clavicle and acromion are marked with a sterile skin marker, as well as the coracoid process and the posterior portal entry site, one thumb's breadth below and medial to the posterior angle of the acromion, as shown before draping in Figure 4.17.

Introducing the needle

A needle is then introduced from the posterior portal entry site, aimed at the surgeon's finger, which has been placed on the coracoid process (Figure 4.18). At this point, it is of benefit to ask for silence in the operating theatre. The assistant then distracts the arm towards the patient's feet, and resistance is felt as the posterior capsule is encountered, followed by a sucking sound as the joint is entered. If there is an effusion within the joint fluid may then escape from the needle showing correct placement (Figure 4.19), but this is rare.

A 50 ml syringe is connected to the needle

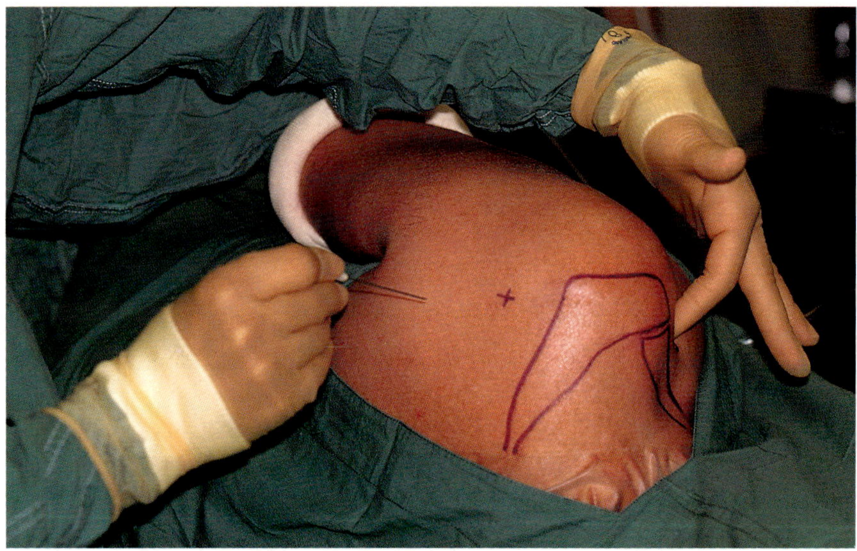

Figure 4.18
A needle is inserted from the posterior portal aimed at the coracoid process.

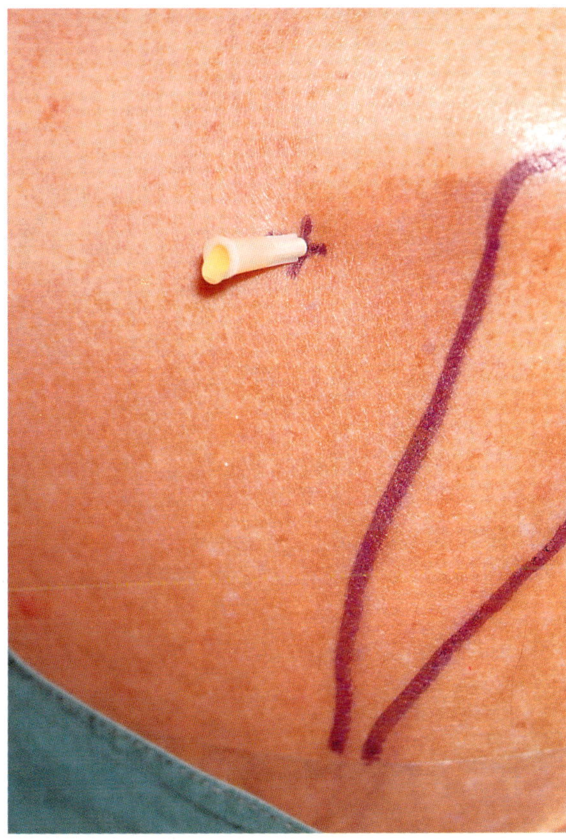

Figure 4.19

A sucking noise is heard as the needle enters the joint. If there is an effusion (which is rare) joint fluid may exit from the needle.

and the joint is prefilled with irrigating fluid (Figure 4.20). We have found that the shoulder will take over 40 ml on average, and up to 70 ml in dislocating shoulders. Free backflow of fluid into the syringe shows correct placement of the needle inside the glenohumeral joint. If there is no backflow, then the needle should be removed and replaced in a better position.

Difficulty can be encountered in prefilling the joint for one of several reasons. The first is inexperience which, of course, is unavoidable. The second is through obliteration of the landmarks by obesity or muscle. A longer needle (spinal needle) is needed. The third reason may be rotator cuff tears, which allow the fluid to pass straight out of the joint into the subacromial space. The last reason is in the stiff painful joint, where the joint is obliterated by synovitis.

The needle and syringe are removed following prefilling. The skin is then punctured using a No 11 surgical blade at the portal site. The incision should follow Langer's lines, and should be long enough to allow the insertion of the arthroscope (Figure 4.21). The sharp trochar and cannula are inserted, following the needle track and aiming for the finger on the coracoid process (Figure 4.22). Fluid is seen to escape from the open side tap showing correct placement (Figure 4.23). The arthroscope is inserted in the place of the trochar, and connected to the irrigation fluid and to the light source (Figure 4.24). The arthroscopic camera is then connected (Figure 4.25), and the camera and light source switched on.

A needle is placed via the anterior portal, the surface marking of which is halfway between the coracoid process and the anterior edge of the acromion, pointing directly towards the arthroscope (Figure 4.26). Entry is confirmed by the outflow of irrigation solution (Figure 4.27). This ensures a free movement of fluid which keeps the joint clear of blood. The difference in calibre of the entry and exit cannulae ensures that pressure is maintained within the joint, as well as establishing a flow.

After the joint has been examined visually (see Chapter 5), extra information is gleaned by palpation. A hook probe needs to be passed from the anterior portal (Figure 4.28). Instruments can be placed into the joint through the anterior portal freehand or through a cannula.

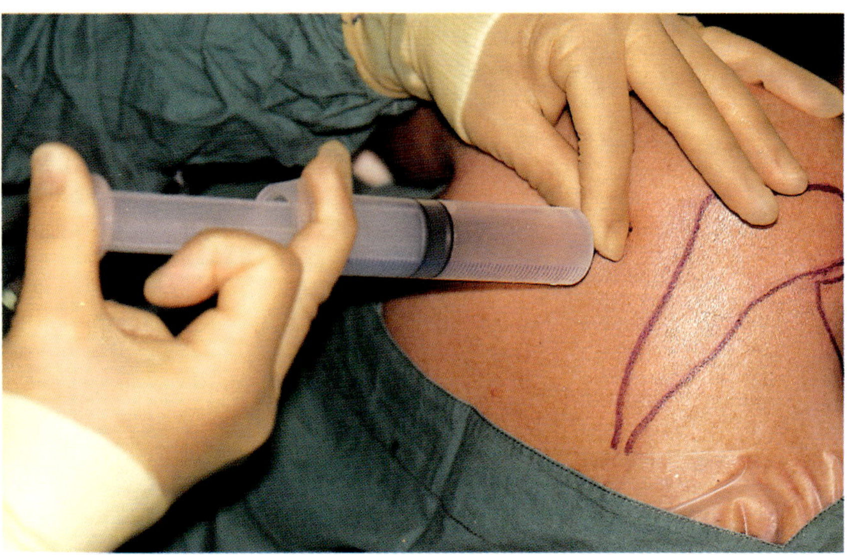

Figure 4.20
The joint is prefilled with sterile irrigation solution. Free backflow shows correct placement.

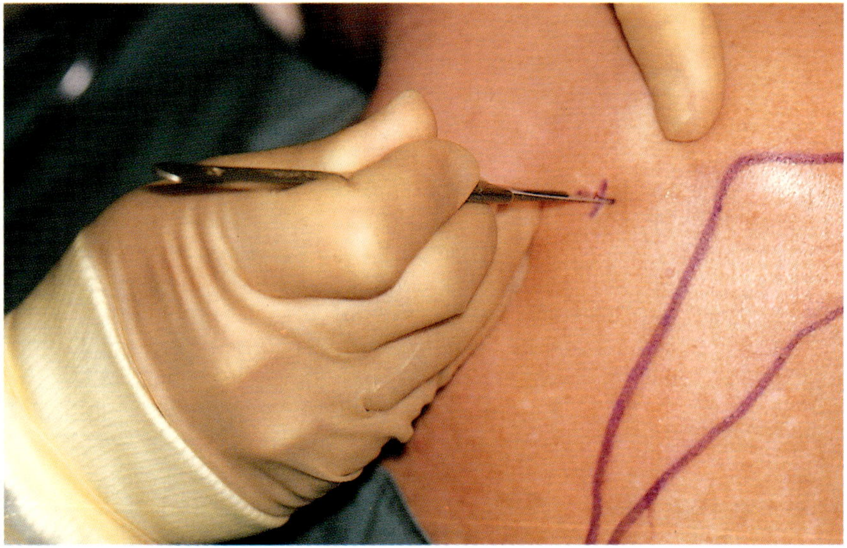

Figure 4.21
An incision along the Langer's line is made at the portal site.

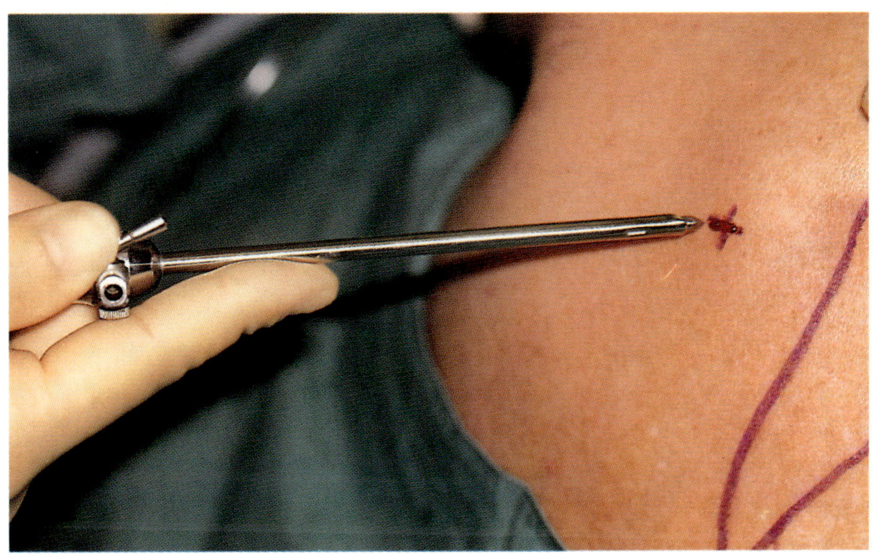

Figure 4.22

The sharp trochar and cannula are then placed following the line of the withdrawn needle.

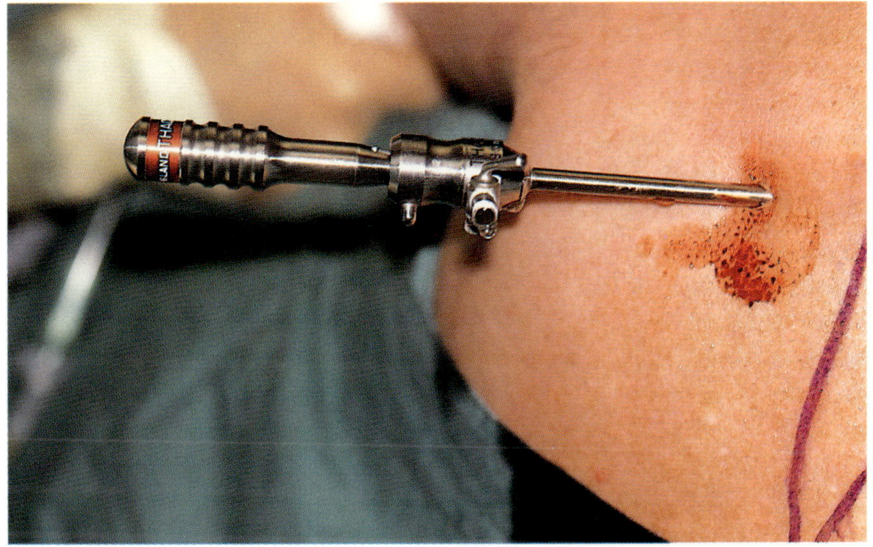

Figure 4.23

Fluid escape from the prefilled joint shows successful placement.

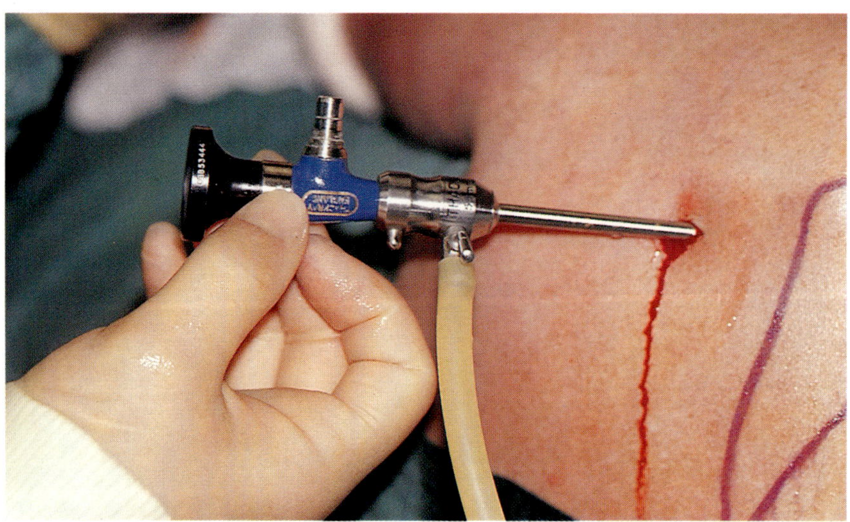

Figure 4.24
The arthroscope is inserted in the cannula, and irrigating fluid and light cable attached.

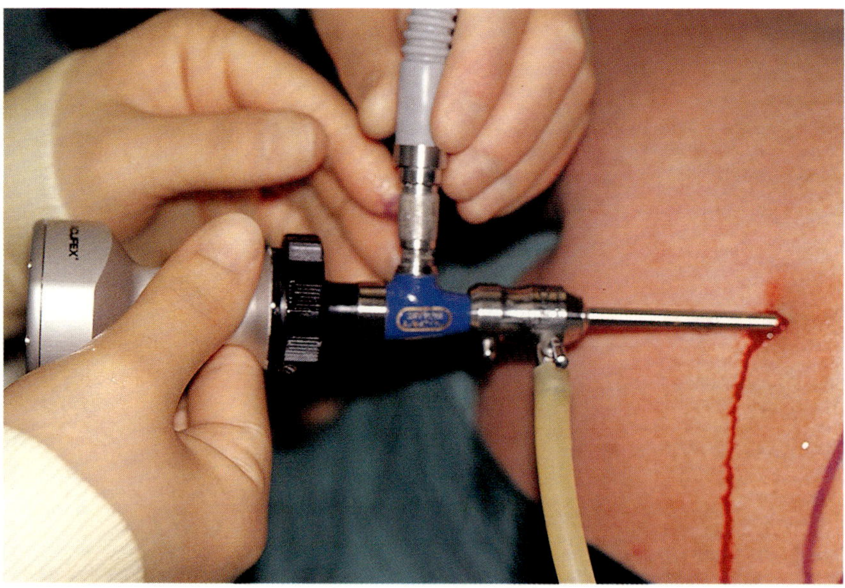

Figure 4.25
The arthroscope camera is finally attached.

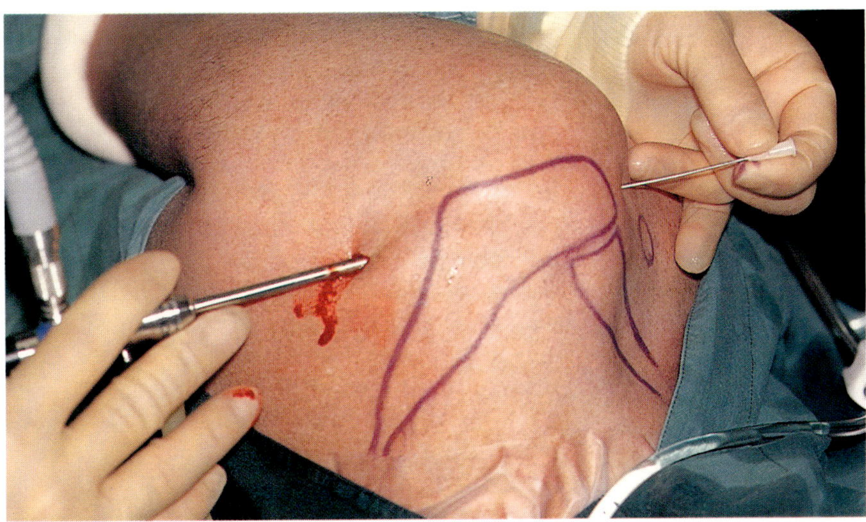

Figure 4.26

A needle is then placed from the anterior portal pointing towards the arthroscope.

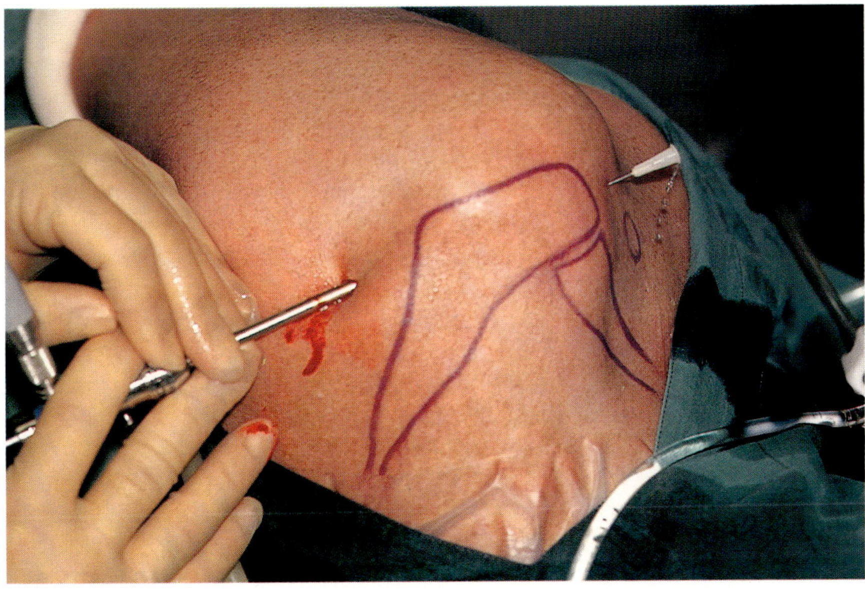

Figure 4.27

Escape of irrigation fluid shows successful placement of the needle, which ensures free flow of fluid and keeps the joint clear of blood.

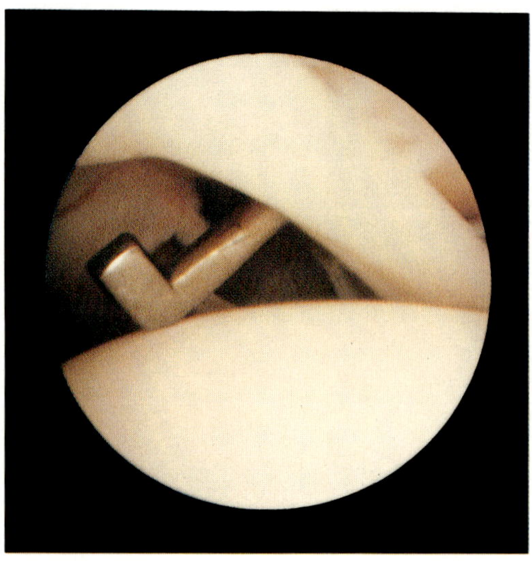

Figure 4.28

A hook probe is then inserted through the anterior portal, using either the inside-out or outside-in technique.

Cannulation

If the instruments are passed freehand, it is best to make a track for them first, by inserting a sharp trochar and cannula down the anterior portal. However, this does not necessarily guarantee that the instruments will follow the track and, if repeated passages are envisaged, then it is best to insert a cannula. There are two methods to pass a cannula, the outside-in technique or the inside-out technique.

Outside-in technique

The arthroscope is brought into the foramen of Weitbrecht and rests on the synovium just above the subscapularis tendon. In the thin patient, the arthroscope can be felt tenting up the soft tissues. Alternatively, the room lights can be lowered, which makes light from the arthroscope visible through the skin, if thin enough. Having marked this site as the insertion site, a 5 mm skin incision is made and the arthroscope backed off so that the plunging sharp cannula does not damage it. The sharp trochar and cannula are inserted, aiming at the site from which the arthroscope tip has been withdrawn. The sharp trochar and cannula are carefully advanced with rotation until joint entry occurs.

Inside-out technique

The inside-out technique is more elegant and was devised by Dr A. Wissinger. The arthroscope is advanced through the foramen of Weitbrecht above the subscapularis tendon, as before, until it rests on the synovium. In this position, the arthroscope is removed, leaving the arthroscope cannula resting on the synovium at the front of the shoulder. A long sharp rod (Wissinger rod) is now passed down the arthroscope cannula from the back of the shoulder and pushed out of the front of the shoulder. As it tents the skin, a 7 mm stab incision is made over it. A cannula is then placed over the rod in front of the shoulder and 'railroaded' down the rod and into the shoulder joint. With both cannulae inside the shoulder joint, one from the posterior portal and the other from the anterior portal, the Wissinger rod is withdrawn and the arthroscope reinserted.

An additional portal can now be used for irrigation (Figure 4.29), the superior or Neviaser portal (see Chapter 3). A Verres needle is placed medial to the acromion in the suprascapular fossa and triangulated to enter the superior part of the joint (Figure 4.30). Some concern has been expressed[10] that this portal may damage the rotator cuff but, in dissections at

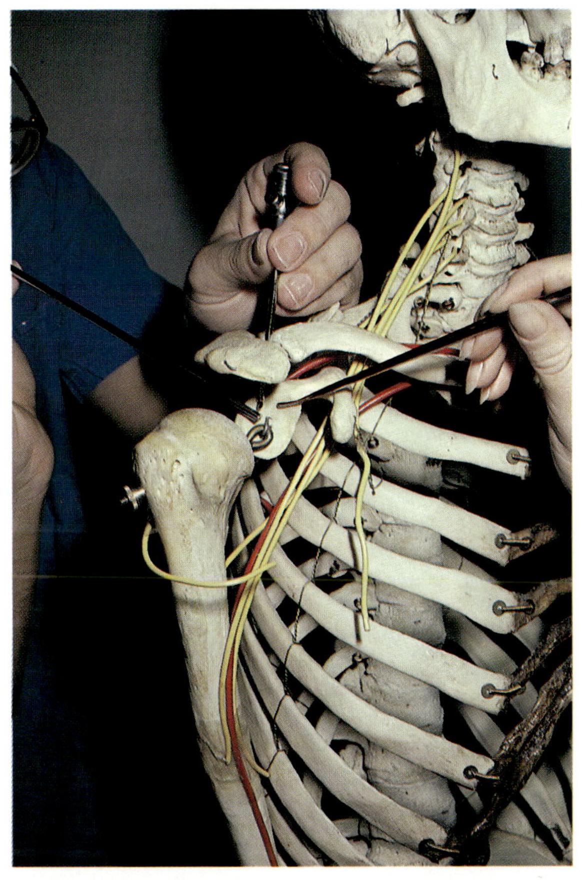

Figure 4.29
The superior portal can be used for irrigation.

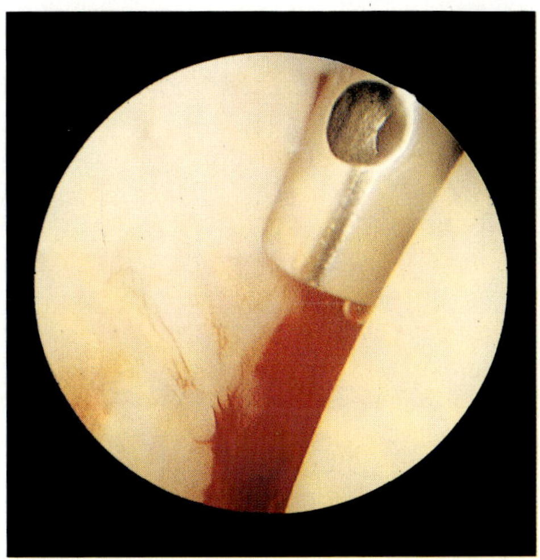

Figure 4.30
The Verres needle can be used to suck blood from the joint.

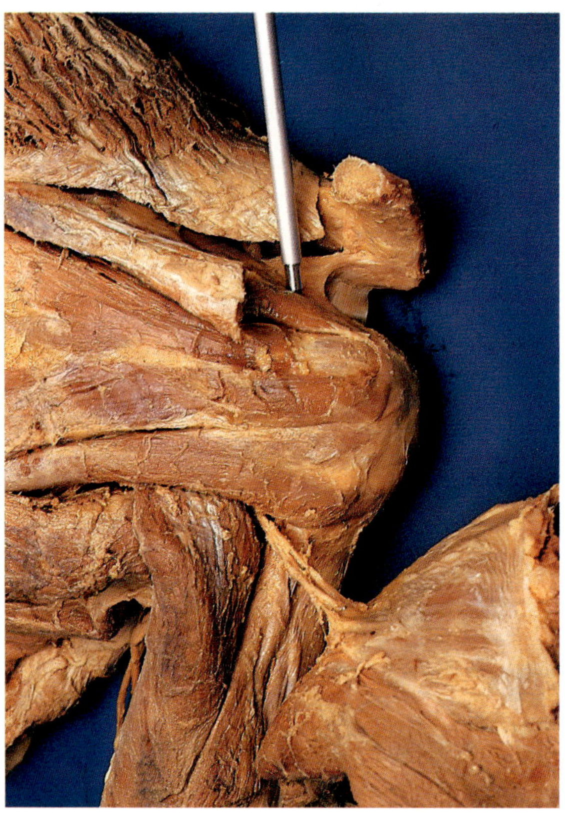

Figure 4.31
The needle passes through muscle and not through tendon.

Nottingham and at other centres, it has been seen that the needle passes through the muscle of supraspinatus and not the tendon (Figure 4.31). The needle can be tucked down in the posterior gutter to avoid instrument clashes. Most procedures can be performed with a two-portal technique, and this third portal is rarely needed.

Bursal endoscopy

After the glenohumeral endoscopy has been performed, it is essential to pass on to the bursal side examination. The arthroscope cannula and sharp trochar are passed either through the same posterior skin incision, or through a separate and slightly higher (cephalad) stab. The sharp trochar is exchanged for the blunt trochar and pushed forward under the acromion until the end of the trochar rests on the coracoacromial ligament. This is helped by the assistant pulling the arm downwards (caudad) with the arm to the side.

The most common error in bursal endoscopy is to fail to enter the bursa, and the reason for

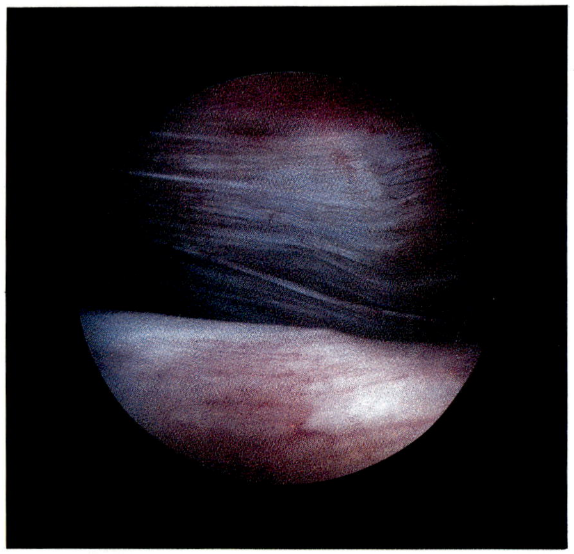

Figure 4.32
If the bursa has successfully been entered, then a large cavity is seen.

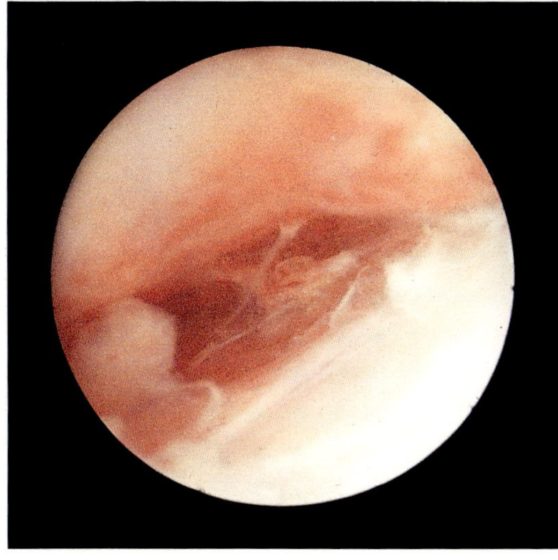

Figure 4.33
If the bursa has not been entered, then the arthroscope is in the subacromial areolar tissue and a 'cobweb' appearance will be seen.

this is simply that most surgeons believe that the subacromial bursa lies under the acromion. In fact it can consistently be entered under the coracoacromial ligament but its extension under the acromion is variable. Bayley (personal communication, 1989) has classified the bursa into three types: where the bursa extends under the anterior one-third of the acromion; where its posterior limit is the anterior edge of the acromion; and where it extends under the anterior two-thirds of the acromion.

In order to enter the bursa every time, therefore, the trochar must be inserted until it is anterior to the acromion and the free lateral edge of the coracoacromial ligament can be flicked on the end of the trochar. The trochar is now withdrawn and the arthroscope inserted. If a large cavity is seen (Figure 4.32), then irrigation may be switched on to expand the bursa. If all that is seen is cobwebs (Figure 4.33), then the bursa has not yet been entered, usually because the cannula is not far enough forward. The irrigation should not be switched on, as this will make entry more difficult. The process is repeated with the cannula further forward.

Orientation within the bursa is more difficult as there are no helpful landmarks like the long head of biceps. It is therefore helpful at this point to insert two needles, one at the anterolateral edge of the acromion and one at the acromioclavicular joint.

Operative portals for subacromial decompression are described in Chapter 8.

5 Normal arthroscopic examination

The normal arthroscopic examination consists of both a glenohumeral arthroscopy and endoscopy of the subacromial space. It is important to devise a consistent routine for shoulder arthroscopy so that the examination is always thorough. This routine examination starts with the tendon of the long head of biceps, moves above it to the cuff, below it and forwards to the anterior capsular structures, down along the anterior labrum into the infraglenoid recess. Finally, the examination goes up along the posterior labrum looking at the back of the humeral head, the bare area, the synovial reflection, the insertion of infraspinatus and the posterior gutter (Figure 5.1).

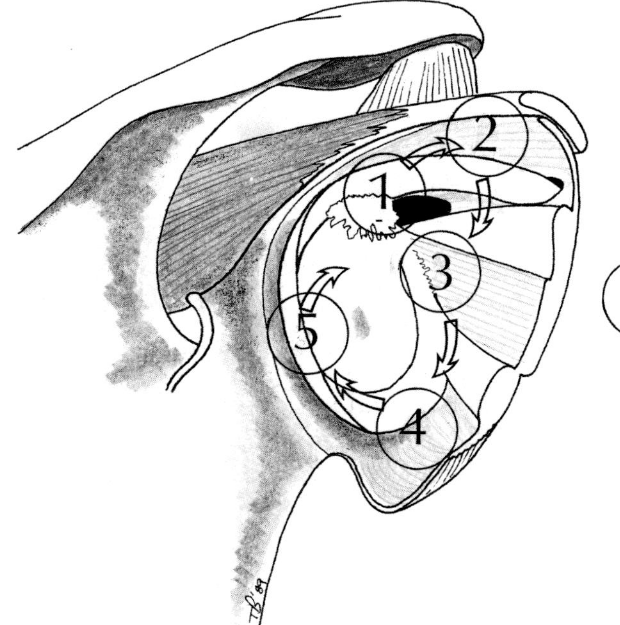

Figure 5.1

A structured method of examining the joint starts with the long head of biceps (1), passes up to look at the cuff (2), then down to the anterior structures (3), down to the inferior recess (4), back up the posterior glenoid (5) and finally looking at the back of the humeral head, the bare area and infraspinatus insertion (6).

Long head of biceps

The primary landmark of shoulder arthroscopy is the tendon of the long head of biceps (LHB). This originates from the supraglenoid tubercle of the scapula but, from the arthroscopist's view, it appears to coalesce with the glenoid labrum, and in particular to flow out from the posterior labrum (Figures 5.2, 5.3 and 5.4). The tendon then arcs its way across the top of the joint, at the same time passing anteriorly over the top of the humeral head (Figures 5.5, 5.6, 5.7 and 5.8). The tendon is round in cross-section as it leaves the labrum, flattens out as it crosses the head, and then becomes rounder as it passes out of the joint below the transverse humeral ligament and into the bicipital canal (Figures 5.9, 5.10, 5.11 and 5.12).

Only one structure can be confused with the long head of biceps – the other intra-articular tendon, the upper border of the tendon of subscapularis. Such different structures could be confused if the arthroscope is inserted too far into the joint. It then comes to rest against the anterior capsular structures and the subscapularis tendon. The arthroscopist's first view will then be a close-up, magnified view of a glistening white tendon, which will be assumed to be the primary landmark, the long head of biceps. As the arthroscope is rotated or pistoned, it soon becomes obvious that the tendon is the subscapularis and the arthroscope should be withdrawn until the biceps flicks into view.

Two variations of the tendon should not be confused for pathological abnormalities. Firstly, the tendon may have a translucent synovial mesentery coming down from the direction of the rotator cuff, which may be vestigial, looking like an adhesion (Figure 5.13), or complete, looking like a transparent sheet (Figure 5.14). Secondly, the tendon may have a cleavage line running down it, as though it were made of two bundles.

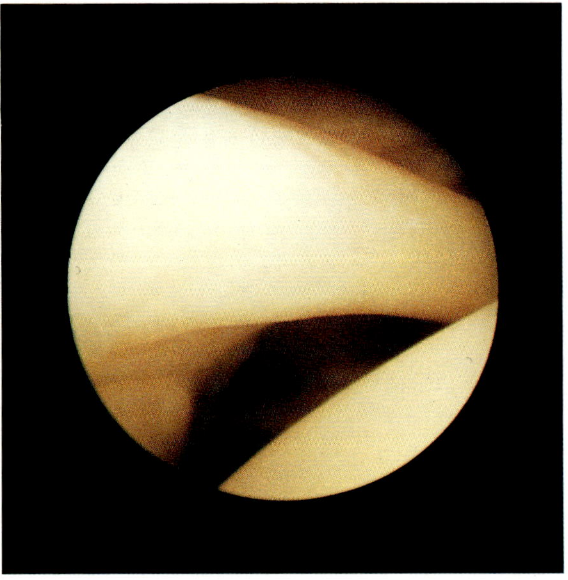

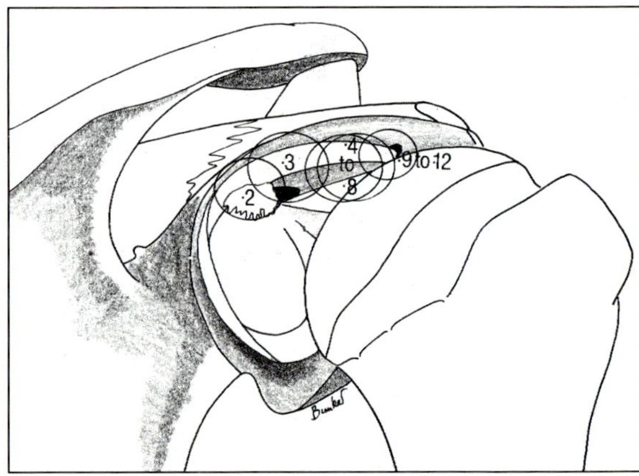

Figure 5.2

The long head of biceps tendon arises from the labrum.

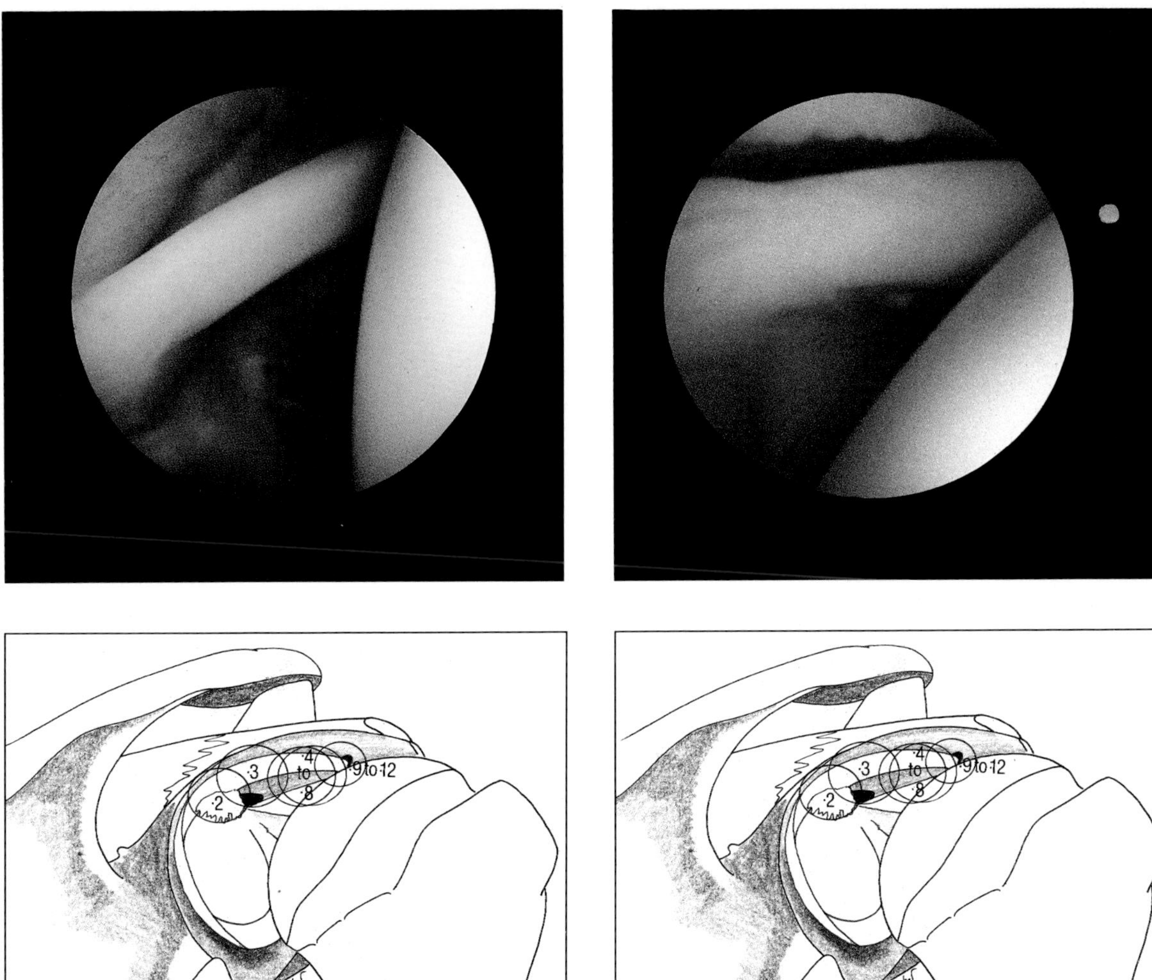

Figures 5.3 to 5.12
Long head of biceps.

Figure 5.4

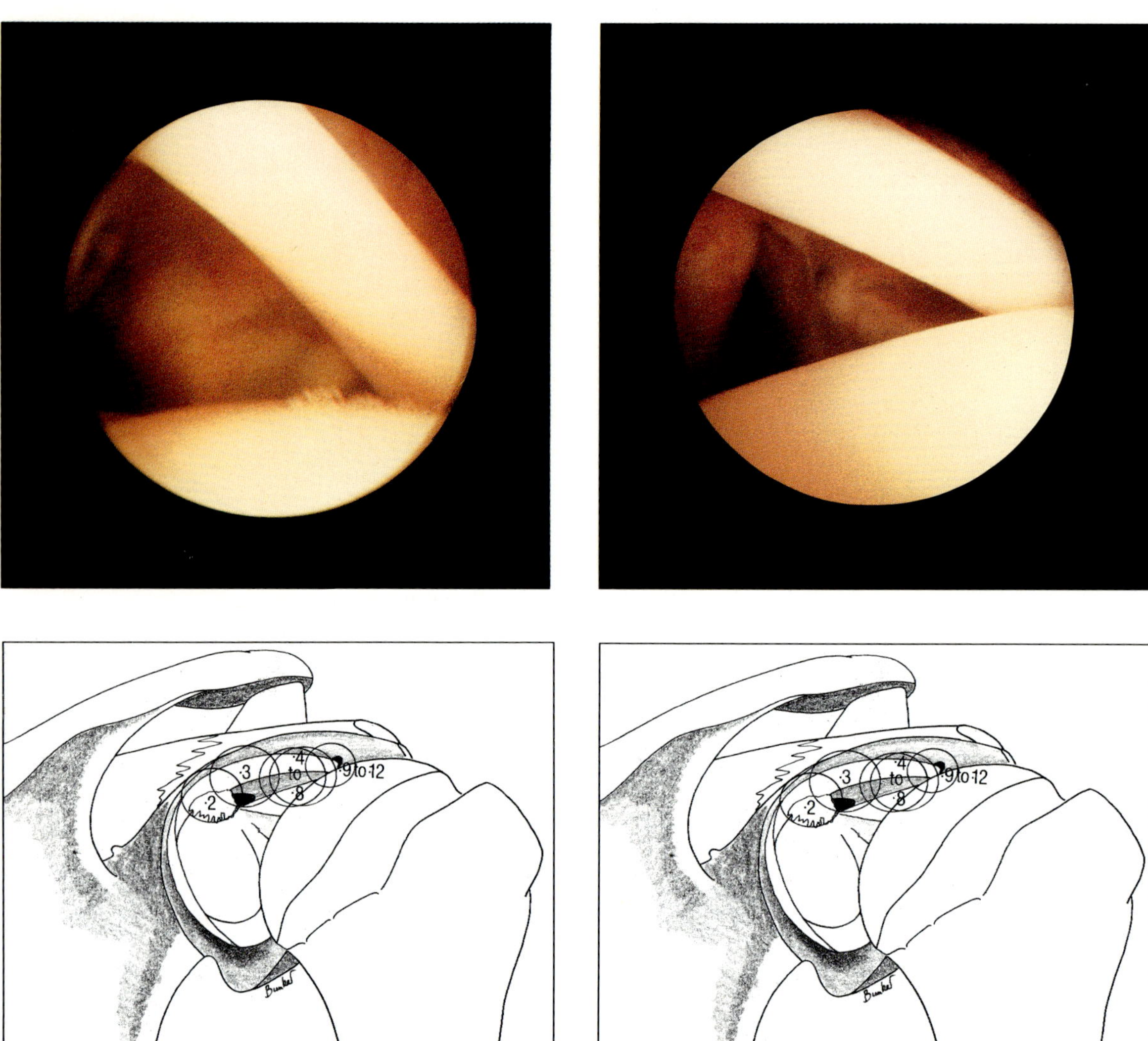

Figure 5.5

Figure 5.6

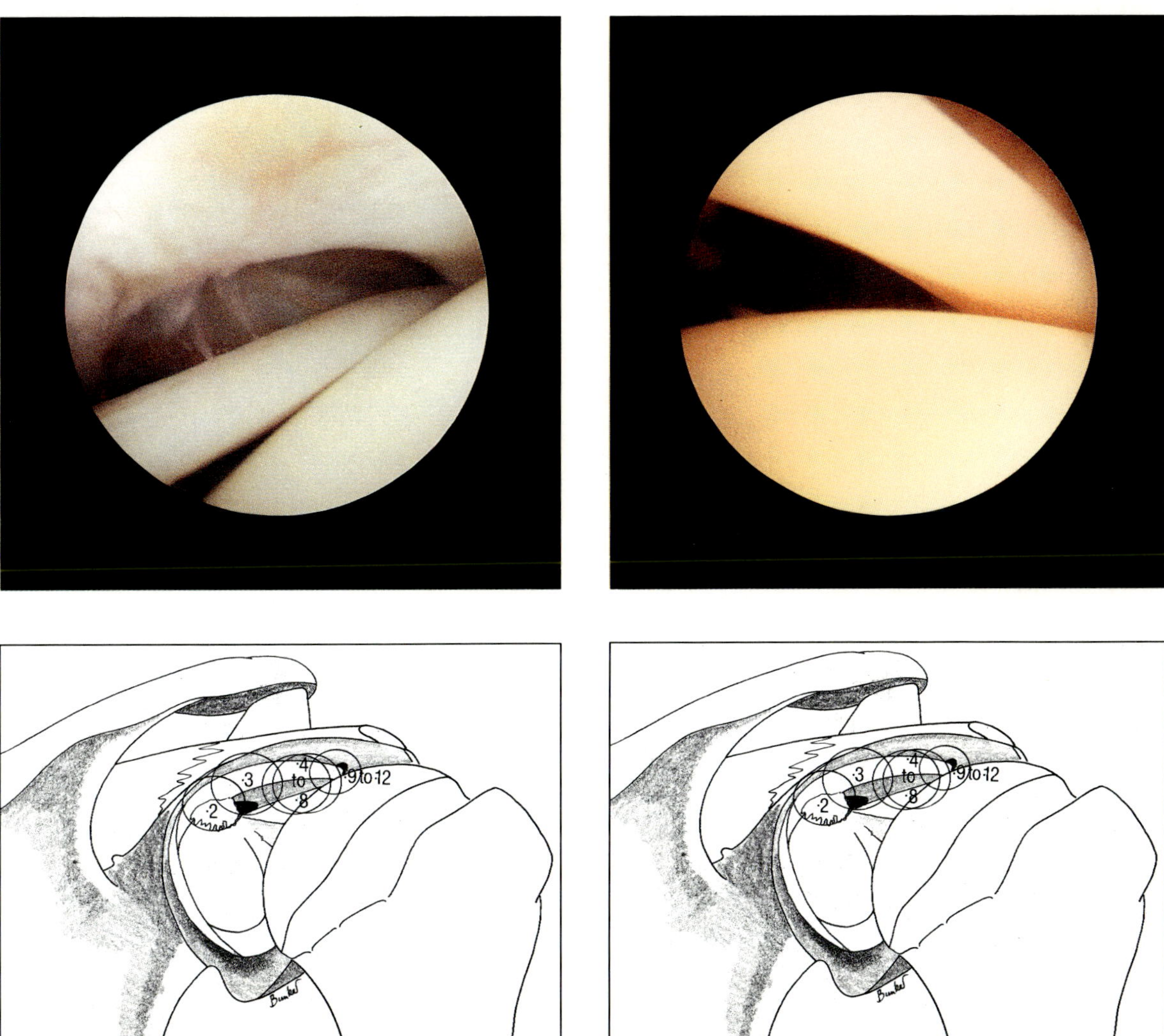

Figure 5.7

Figure 5.8

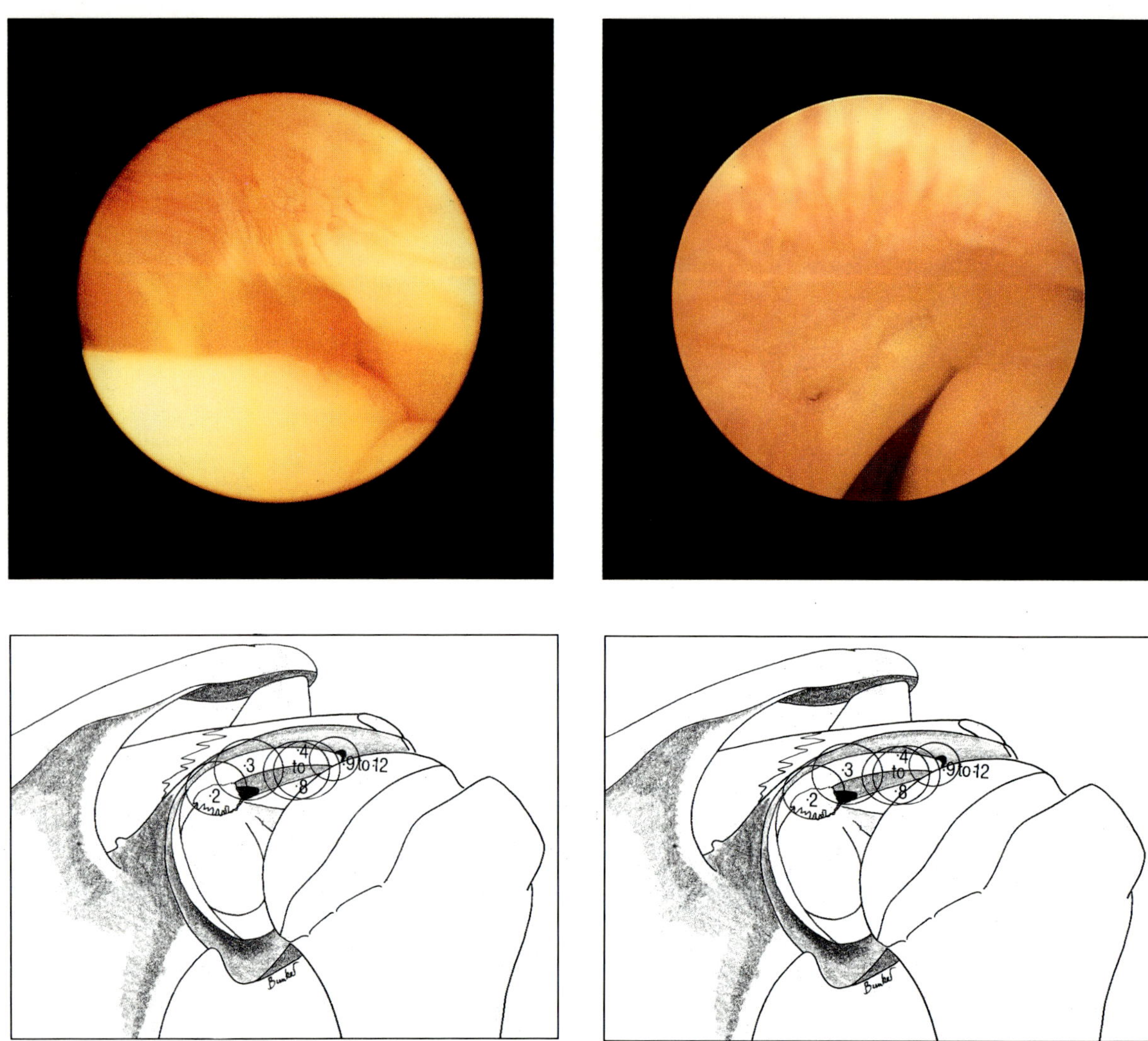

Figure 5.9

Figure 5.10

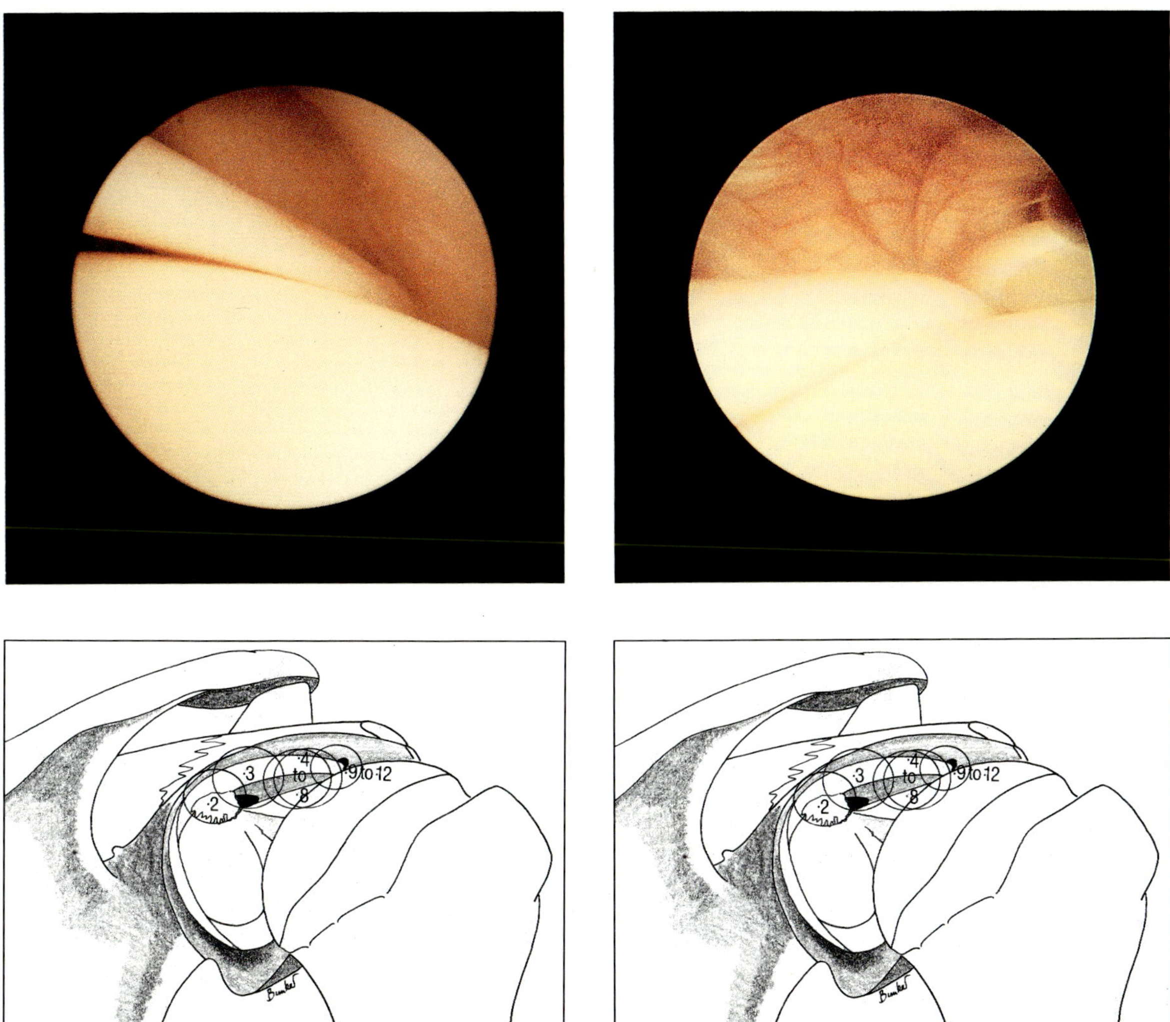

Figure 5.11

Figure 5.12

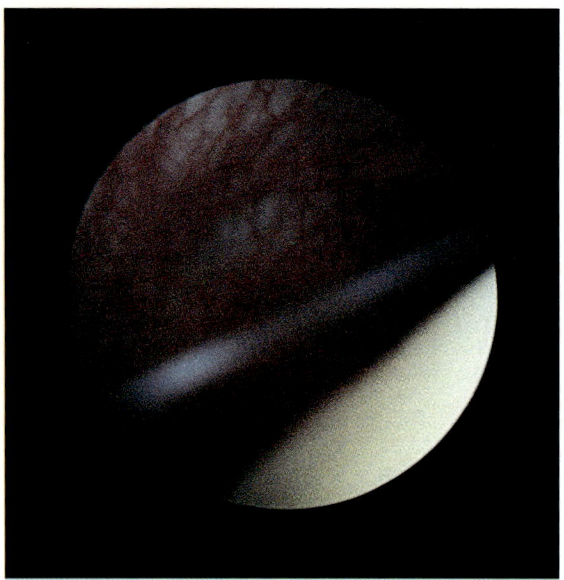

Figure 5.13

Occasionally there is a synovial adhesion to the long head of biceps tendon.

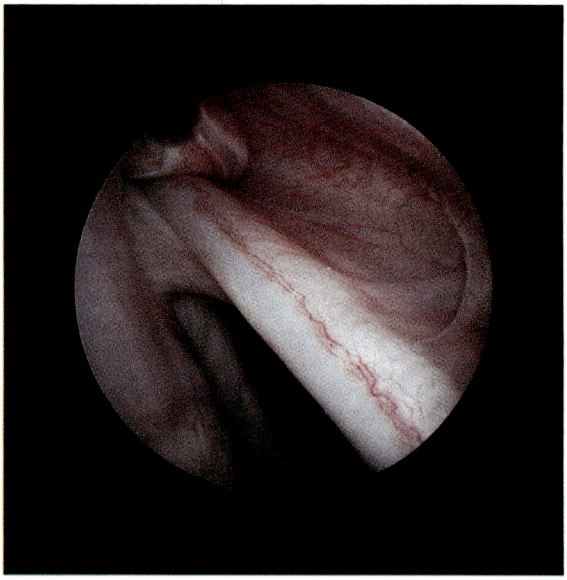

Figure 5.14

Rarely the synovium may infold the biceps tendon like a mesentery.

Rotator cuff

Keeping to the routine, the next part of the joint to inspect is the rotator cuff. The arthroscope is passed over the top of the long head of biceps and carefully withdrawn with rotation to get a good view of the rotator cuff (Figure 5.15). It is important not to withdraw so far that the arthroscope comes out of the joint, which is easily done at this point. Care should be taken to visualize correctly the rotator cuff that is now seen, and not the undersurface of the acromion. This may be mistakenly visualized through a massive rotator cuff tear, where the edges of the tear have retracted out of view (Figure 5.16). The arthroscope is now passed along the fibres of the rotator cuff and the humerus internally rotated to examine the insertion of the cuff (Figure 5.17). This is the area where cuff tears start, and small cuff tears could be missed. Often the tendon appears to thin out in a crescentic line at the musculotendinous junction, and this should not be mistaken for a tear.

Having visualized the intra-articular portion of supraspinatus, the arthroscope is passed below the long head of biceps and into the intra-articular triangle.[1] This is the triangle bounded above by the long head of biceps, medially by the glenoid and anterosuperior labrum, and is the guide to the anterior capsular structures.

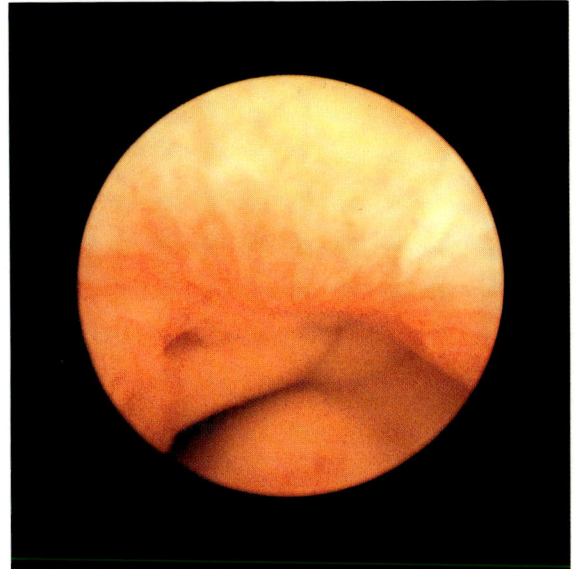

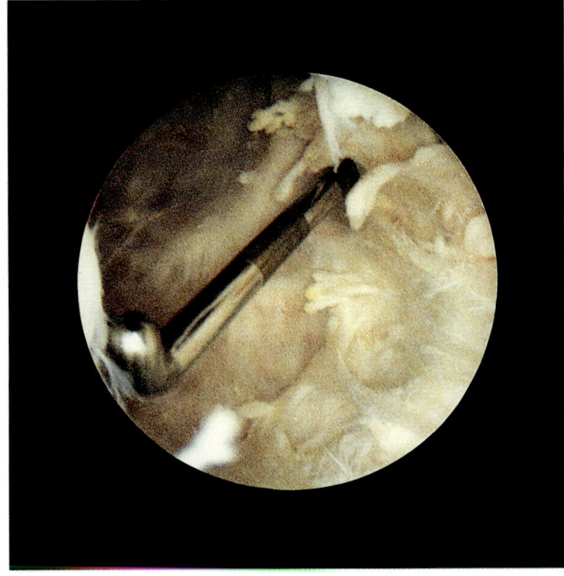

Figure 5.16

Massive rotator cuff tear. The undersurface of the acromion is seen directly, there is no cuff, nor can the retracted cuff edges be seen.

Figure 5.15

Normal rotator cuff above the biceps.

Subscapularis tendon

The most obvious structure is the subscapularis tendon (Figure 5.18), the secondary landmark of shoulder arthroscopy. The superior border is quite clearly intra-articular, lying in a synovial recess between the superior glenohumeral and middle glenohumeral ligaments. This synovial recess is a constant anatomical feature[2] – the opening to what used to be termed the subscapularis bursa. This is a misnomer for a bursa is, by definition, a synovial sac containing synovial fluid which does not connect with a joint. The subscapularis recess is actually a constant synovial outpouching, as is the suprapatellar pouch in the knee, and the term

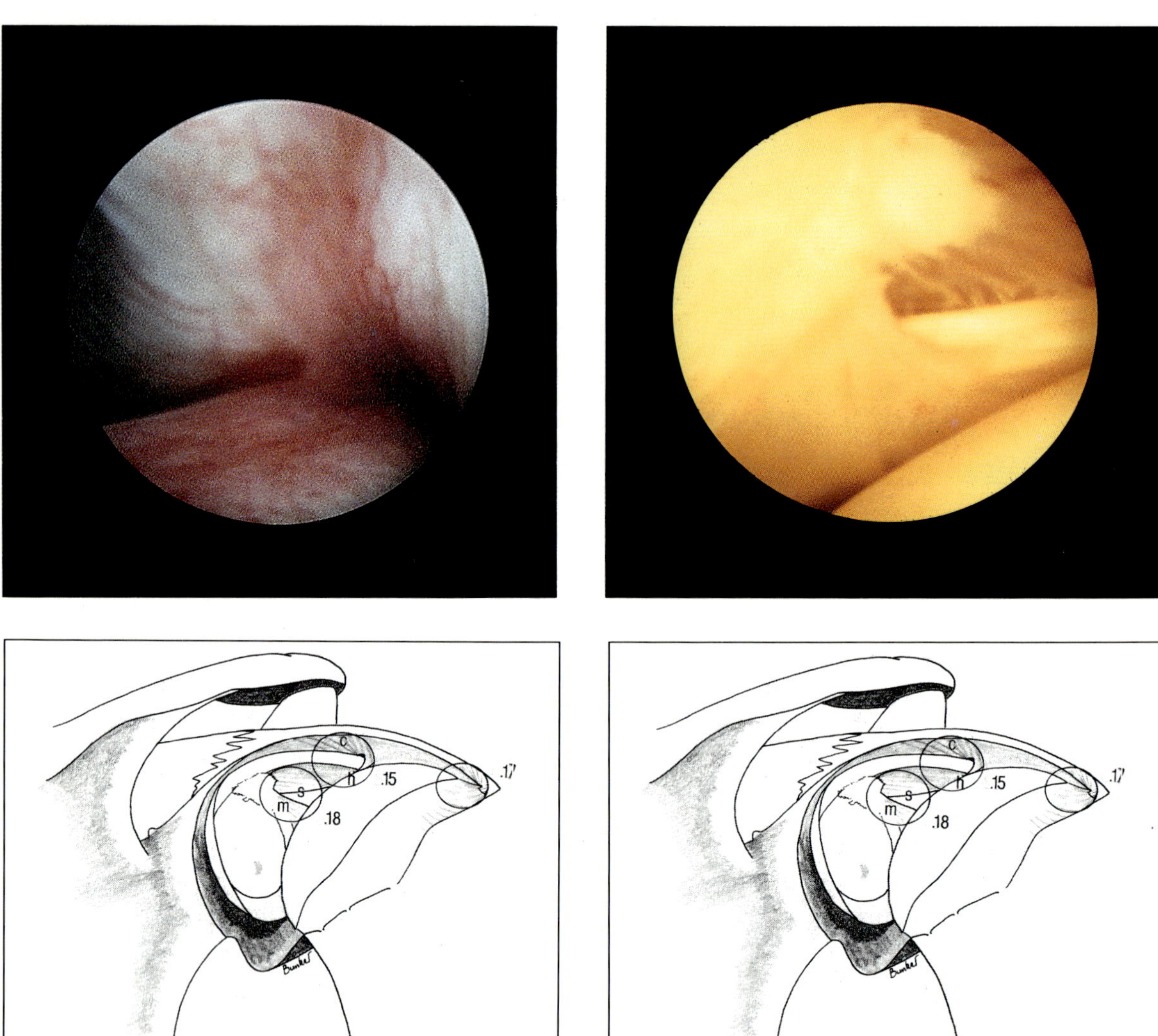

Figure 5.17

The insertion of the rotator cuff.

Figure 5.18

Subscapularis (s) appearing from behind the middle glenohumeral ligament (m).

'subscapularis bursa' should be dropped in favour of 'subscapularis recess' or pouch. The entrance to the subscapularis recess is called the foramen of Weitbrecht. In the lateral decubitus position used for shoulder arthroscopy, the subscapularis recess is the lowermost part of the joint, and is favoured by gravity as a hiding place for loose bodies.

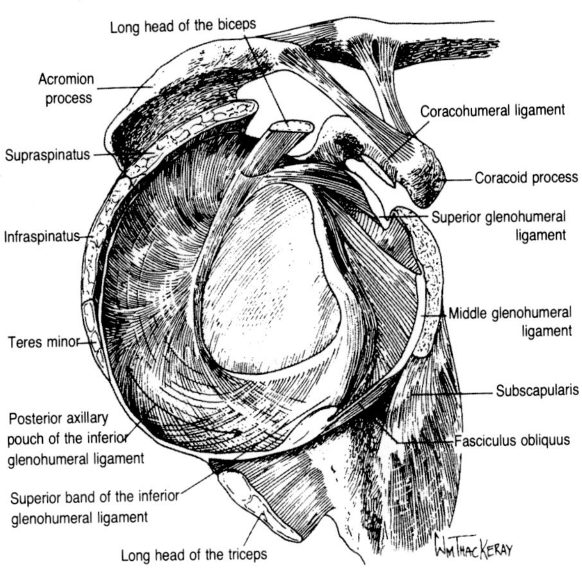

Figure 5.19

Anatomy of the glenohumeral ligaments according to Turkel et al. (From Turkel SJ, Panio MW, Marshall JL et al, Stabilizing mechanisms preventing anterior dislocation of the glenohumeral joint, *J Bone Joint Surg* (1981) **63A** 1208–17.)

Glenohumeral ligaments

The glenohumeral ligaments are always a source of great interest, as such a high proportion of shoulder disability is related to anterior dislocation or subluxation. The anterior shoulder capsule was described by Galen, but the three glenohumeral ligaments were only described and named in the last century. The importance of these ligaments has really only come to the fore with the advent of shoulder arthroscopy, as they are far more obvious from inside the joint than from outside. A great amount has been written about the glenohumeral ligaments and their importance in recurrent dislocation, but for those interested in shoulder arthroscopy the paper of Turkel et al[3] is essential reading (Figure 5.19).

The superior glenohumeral ligament lies above the subscapularis recess and makes up the superior margin of the foramen of Wietbrecht. This ligament is often partially hidden by the long head of biceps when arthroscoping from the posterior portal (Figure 5.20).

The middle glenohumeral ligament varies from a thin membranous structure (Figure 5.21) to a thick ligament, although its position is constant. The middle glenohumeral ligament can always be found crossing obliquely down across the subscapularis bursa and hiding all but the upper leading edge of the tendon from view (Figure 5.22).

The inferior glenohumeral ligament is the strongest and most important of the glenohumeral ligaments. The superior band is constant and can be seen passing downwards and outwards beneath the middle glenohumeral ligament (Figures 5.23 and 5.24). Often the inferior glenohumeral ligament can distinctly be seen as a prolongation of the anterior labrum (Figure 5.25). O'Brien and Warren[4] have looked in detail at the gross and microscopical nature of this ligament. They liken the ligament to a hammock, strung between the glenoid and the humeral head (Figure 5.26). The two ropes holding the hammock are the anterior superior band and, at the back, the posterior superior band. They have shown that the ligament thickens at these two points and that the configuration of the collagen bundles varies within the ligament, passing coronally between the glenoid and the humerus in the thickened

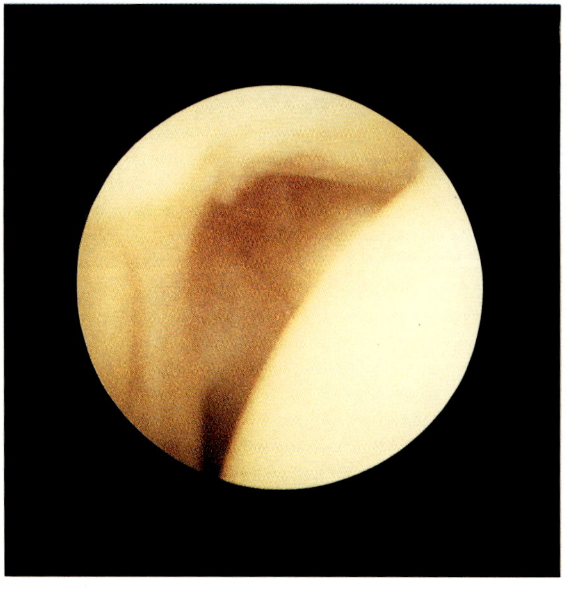

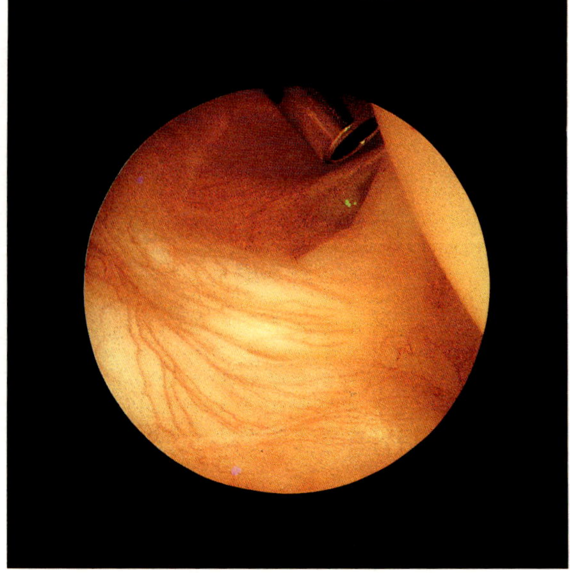

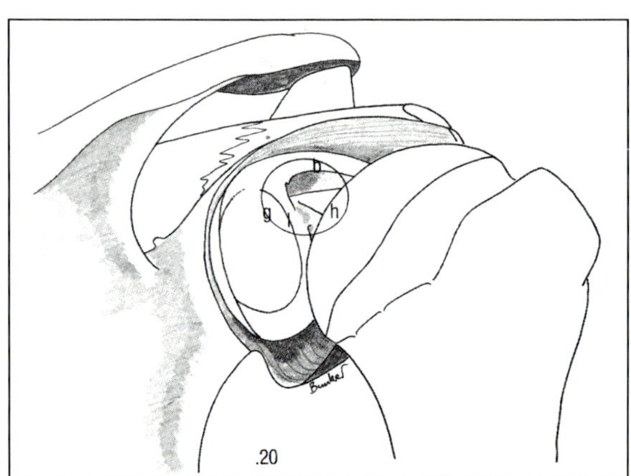

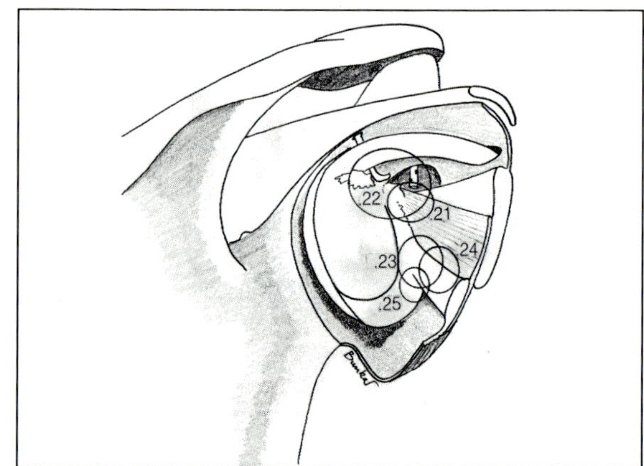

Figure 5.20

The superior glenohumeral ligament is often hidden by the long head of the biceps tendon. b = biceps, h = humerus, l = labrum, g = glenoid.

Figure 5.21

The middle glenohumeral ligament may be thin and wispy.

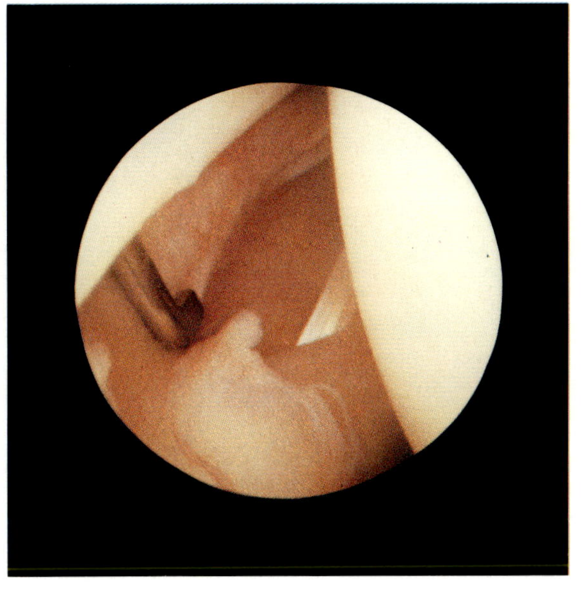

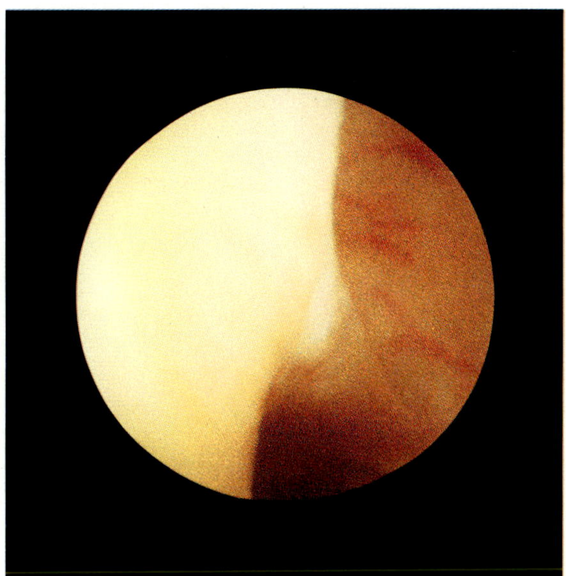

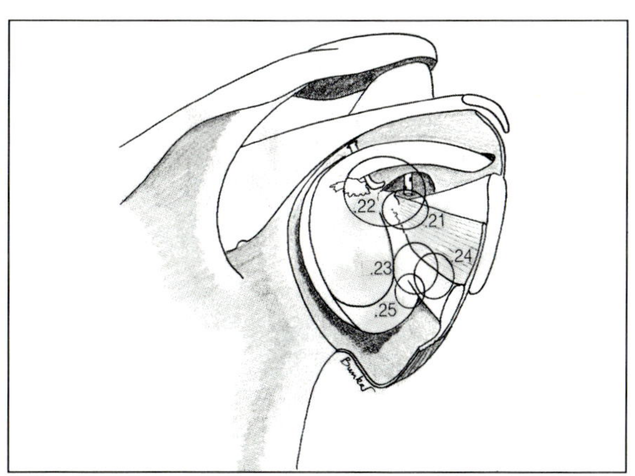

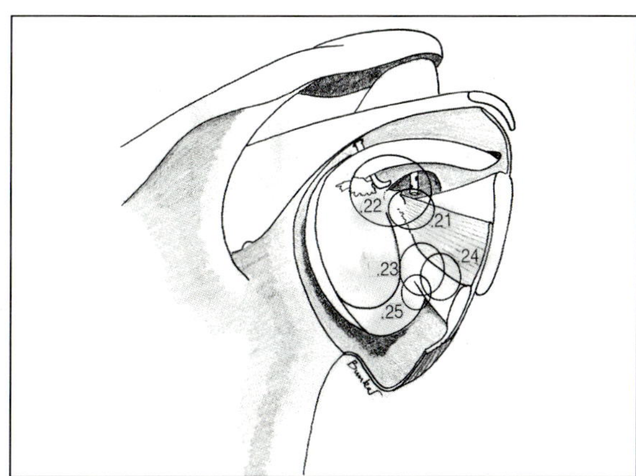

Figure 5.22

Alternatively, the middle glenohumeral ligament may be thick.

Figures 5.23, 5.24 and 5.25

The superior band of the inferior glenohumeral ligament originates from the labrum.

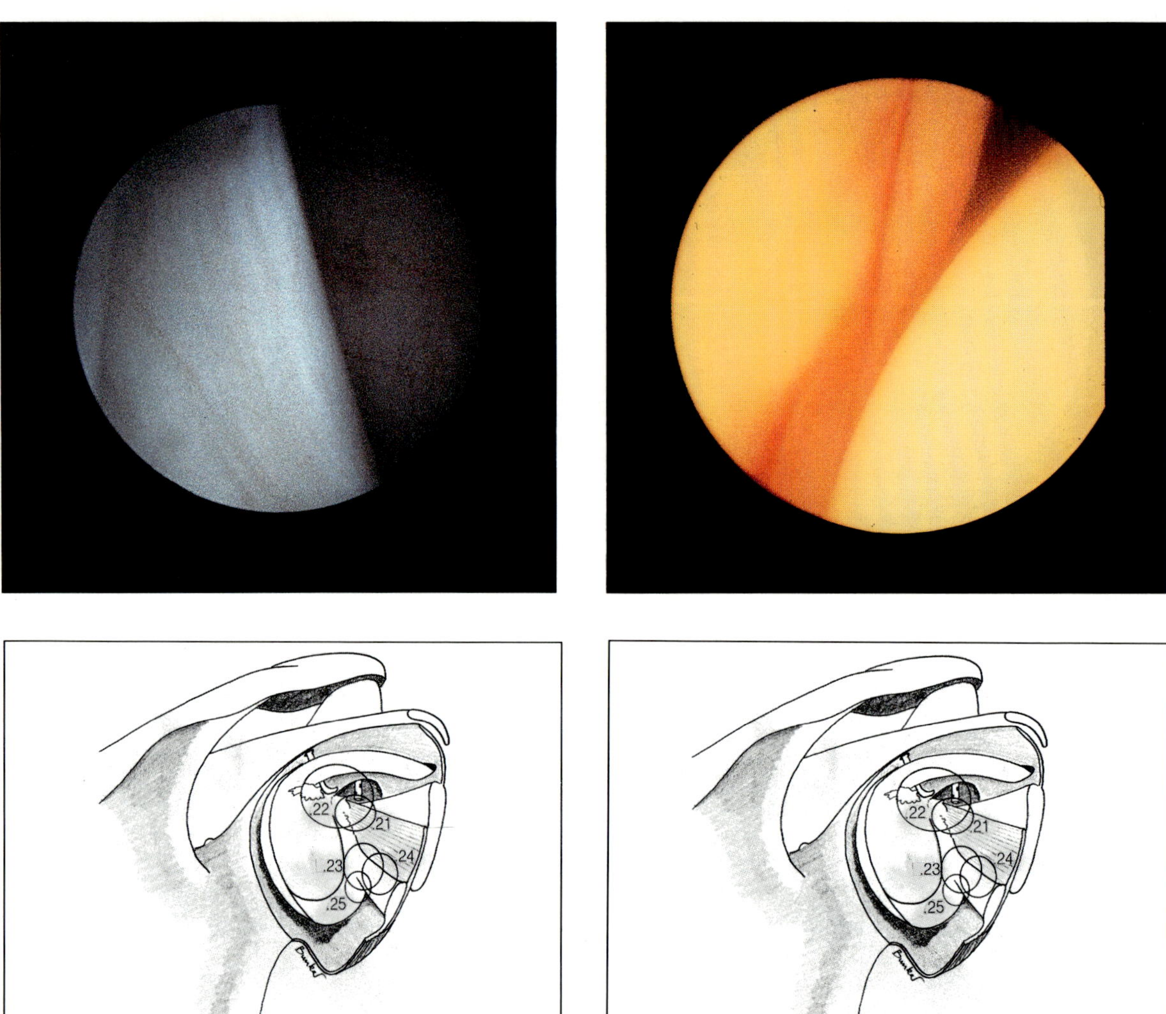

Figure 5.24

Figure 5.25

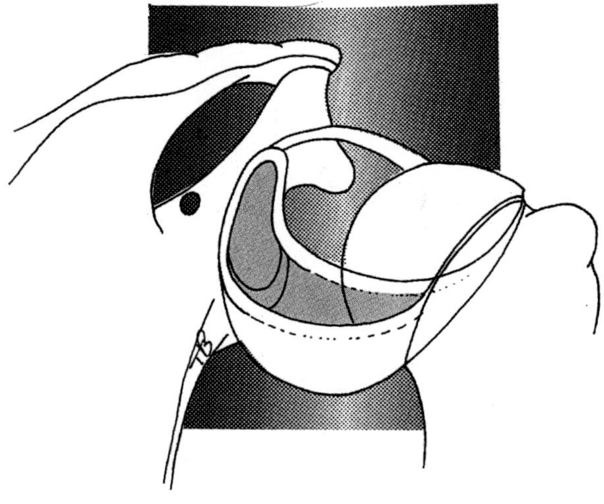

Figure 5.26

The inferior glenohumeral ligament can be likened to a hammock, the superior bands at the front and the back being the ropes which hold up the hammock.

superior bands, and sagittally in the substance of the ligament between these bands. So it is the latter that makes up the infraglenoid recess which, with the arm at the side, is a capacious space (Figures 5.27, 5.28 and 5.29).

The arthroscope is now rotated within the infraglenoid recess to see the synovial reflection on the humeral neck. The arthroscope is now withdrawn gradually with rotation, for it is easy to withdraw too far at this point and exit the joint through the puncture point in the posterior capsule. As the arthroscope is rotated, so the posterior glenoid labrum can be seen (Figures 5.30, 5.31 and 5.32) and behind it the posterior gutter or synovial recess. As the arthroscope is rotated in the other direction, so the posterior surface of the humeral head is observed. At this point, it is important to look carefully at the synovial reflection, or so-called bare area of the humeral head (Figures 5.33 and 5.34) as it is easy for the inexpert arthroscopist to mistake this for a Hill–Sachs lesion. The difference is that the bare area coalesces with the synovial reflection on the neck of the humerus, whereas a Hill–Sachs lesion has a ridge of bone or cartilage between it and the bare area. The bare area often has small pits or holes in it which can clearly be seen, and the junction between it and the articular surface of the head is more normal than the rounded-off fracture of a Hill–Sachs lesion. Further withdrawal and rotation brings the arthroscope back into the triangle between the long head of biceps, the humeral head and the glenoid.

Hook probe

As with arthroscopy of the knee, further tactile information can now be gleaned by the use of a hook probe. This is more difficult to insert than in the knee, and when learning it is often easier to start probing with a 14- or 12-gauge needle (Figure 5.35), or a Verres needle (Figure 5.36). The needle will cause less damage on insertion, and will also establish a flow through the joint. This clears any blood that may at this stage have started to obscure vision. If a hook probe is used it often helps to make a track with a sharp obturator and cannula from the anterior portal and then pass the hook down this track.

Probing the glenoid labrum may show a Bankart lesion, or confirm one, if suspected. The ligaments can be probed in turn and then the long head of biceps and the superior cuff can be palpated.

On completion of the examination, the joint is thoroughly flushed through, the fluid removed from the shoulder, and the probe and arthroscope withdrawn.

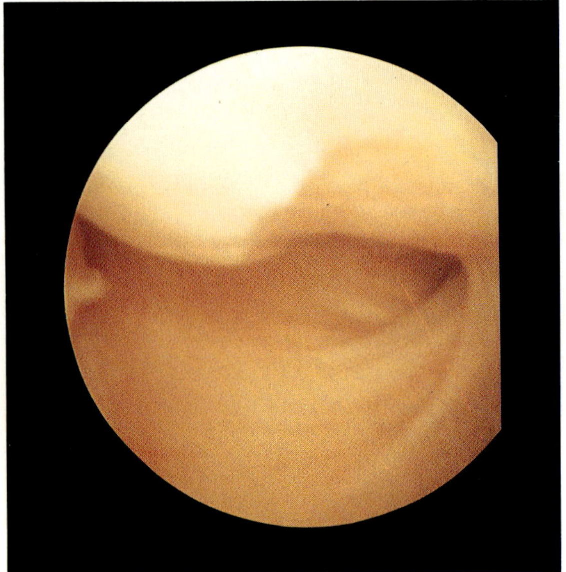

Figure 5.27

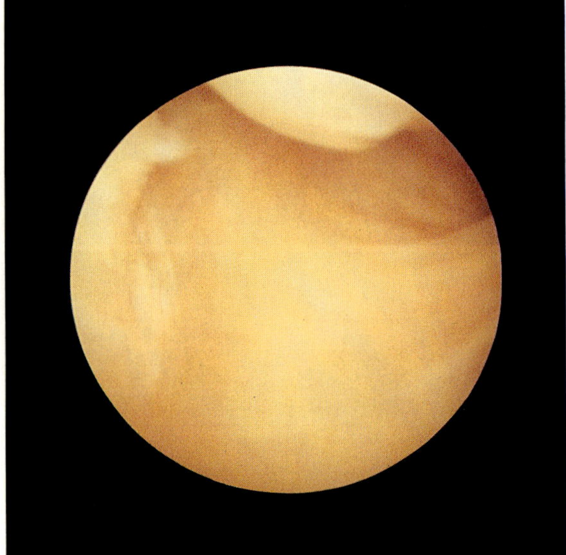

Figure 5.28

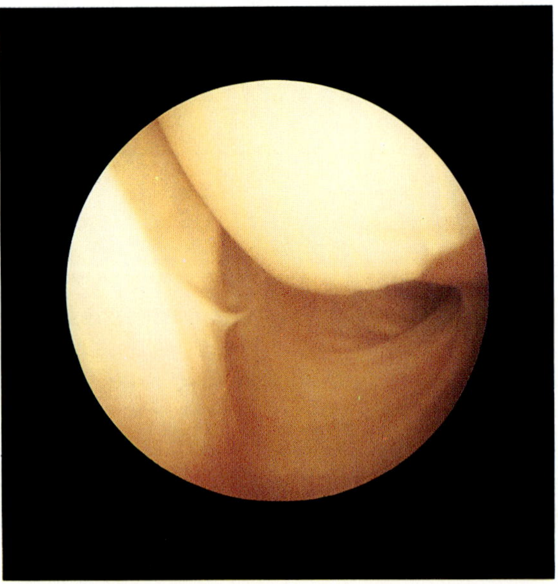

Figures 5.27, 5.28 and 5.29

The infraglenoid recess is a capacious space below the humeral neck.

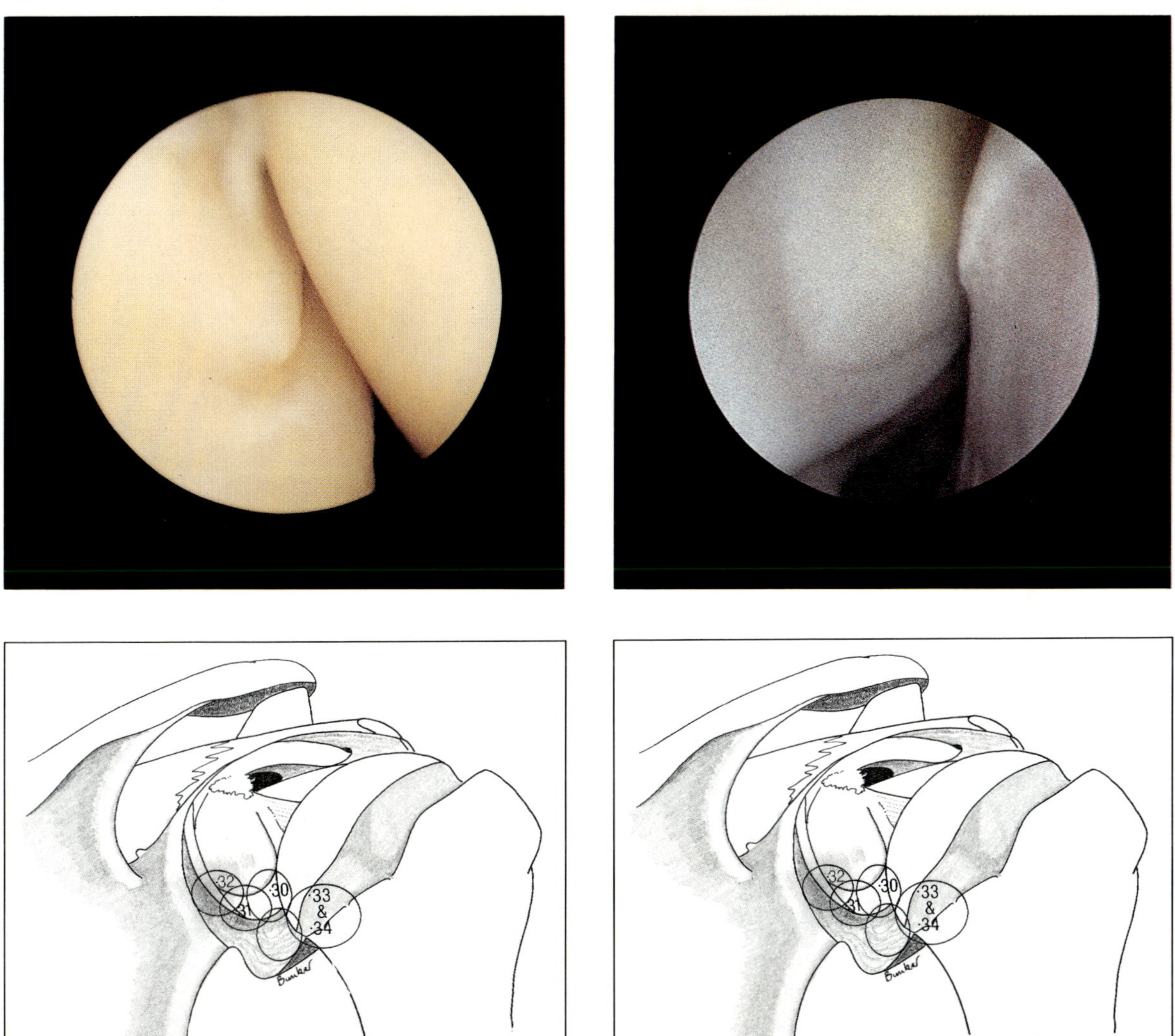

Figures 5.30, 5.31 and 5.32

The inferior and posterior glenoid labrum.

Figure 5.31

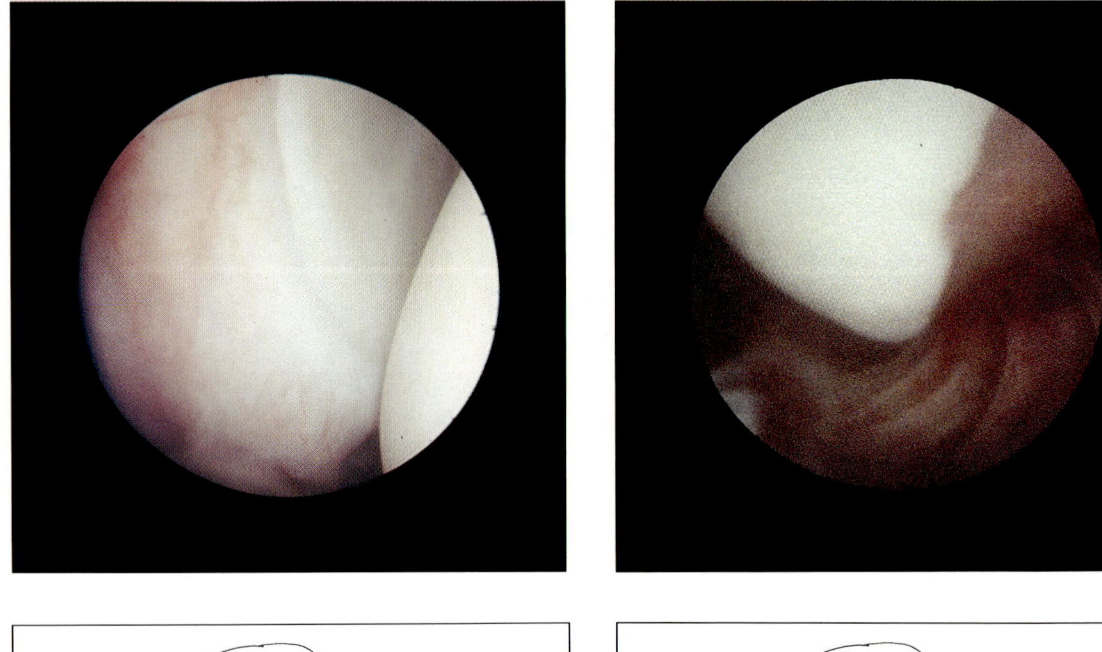

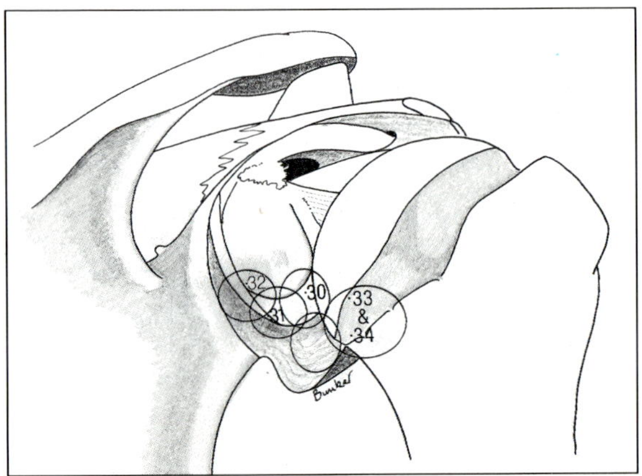

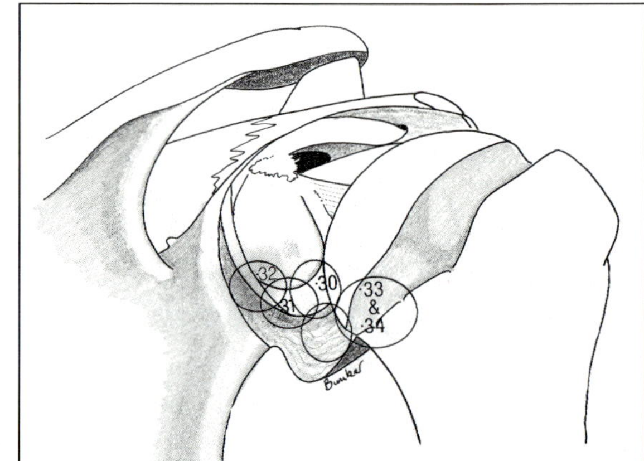

Figure 5.32

Figures 5.33 and 5.34
The bare area of the humerus.

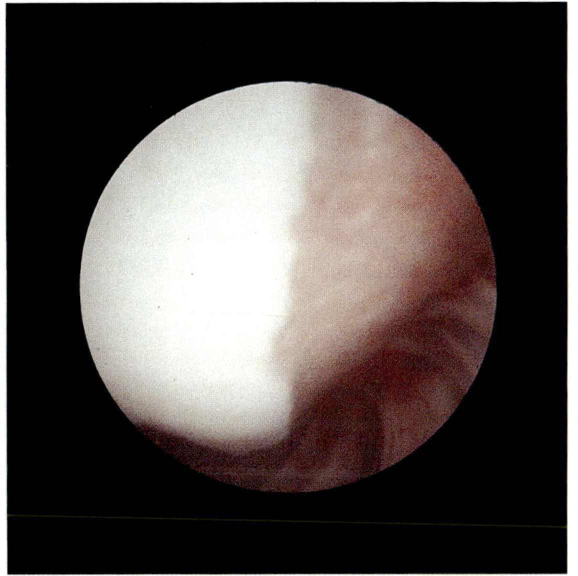

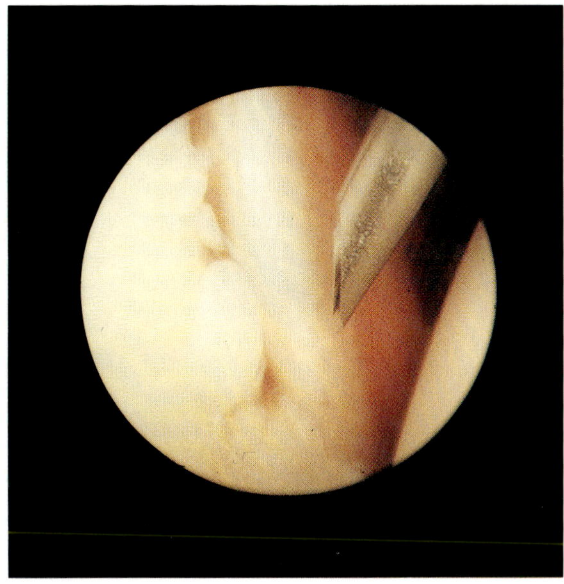

Figure 5.35
A needle used as a probe.

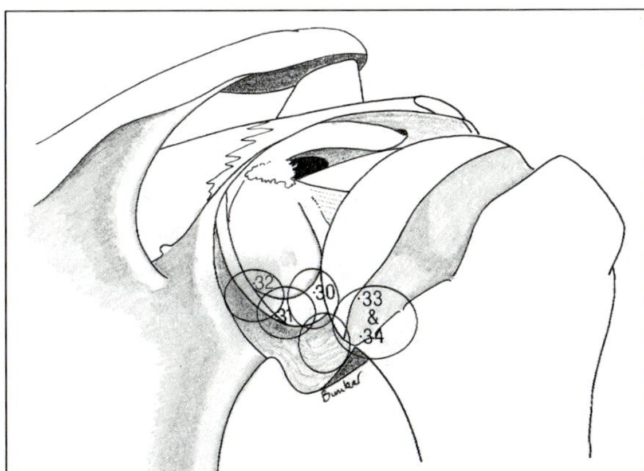

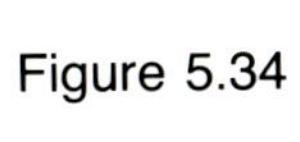

Figure 5.34

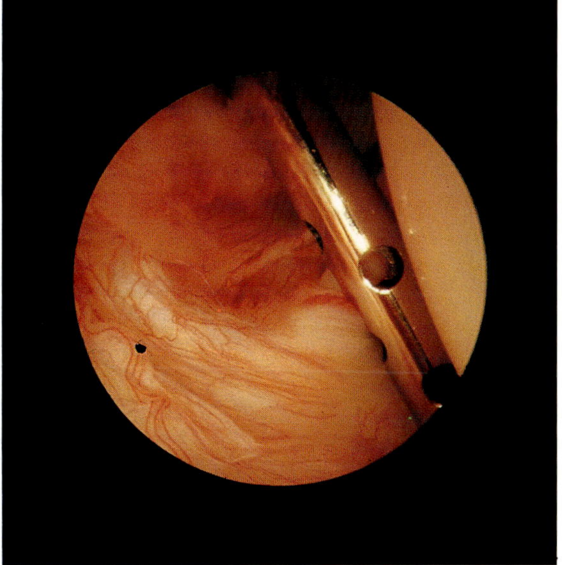

Figure 5.36
Verres needle used as a probe.

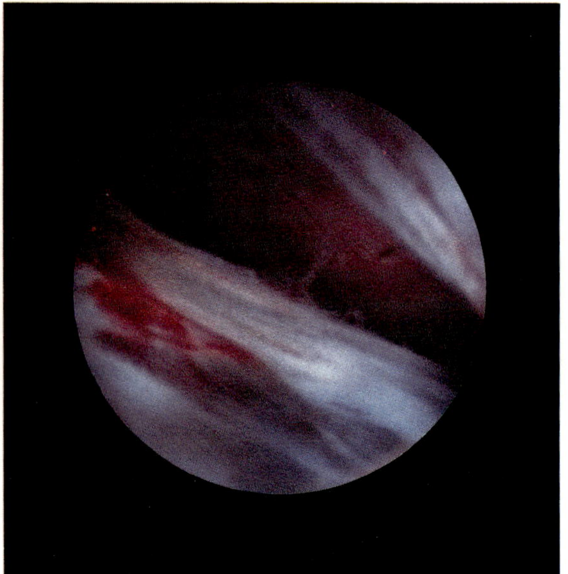

Figure 5.37
If the arthroscope is in the subacromial areolar tissue, posterior to the bursa, the space will seem to be full of 'cobwebs'.

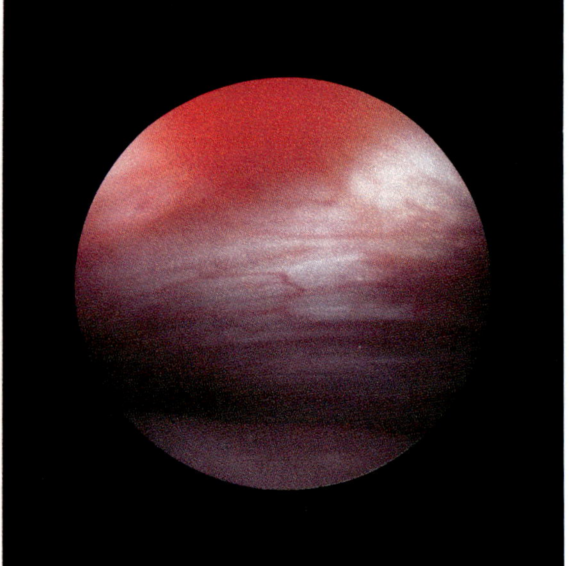

Figure 5.38
The bursa, when successfully entered, is a large space.

Bursoscopy

Examination of the bursa, or bursoscopy, is more difficult than glenohumeral arthroscopy, but should be a routine part of the examination, particularly if clinically the patient has a painful arc of motion. The arthroscope is reinserted through the posterior portal with a blunt obturator inserted. The cannula and trochar are directed just under the acromion.

The most common fault of the inexperienced arthroscopist is failure to enter the bursa. In order to do this, the arm should be alongside the body, for this will increase the potential space available. Distraction of the arm is then applied in the direction of the feet, and the key is to push the cannula until the coracoacromial ligament can be felt on the tip of the blunt trochar. The trochar is moved from side to side and the coracoacromial ligament can be felt to

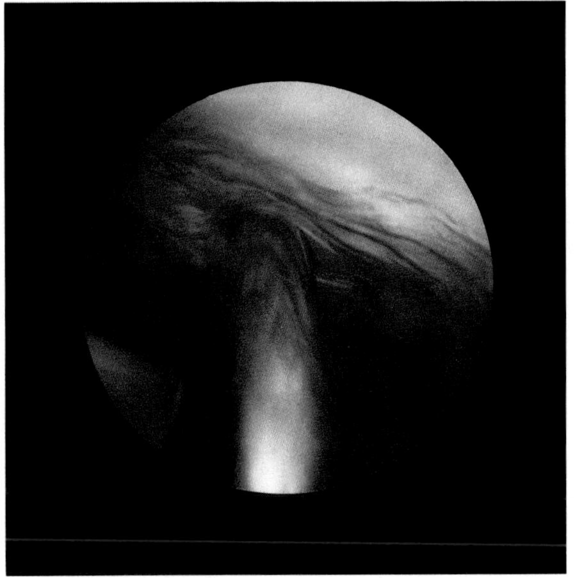

Figure 5.39
Orientation within the bursa is aided by placing needles to each side of the coracoacromial ligament, at the anterior edge of the acromion.

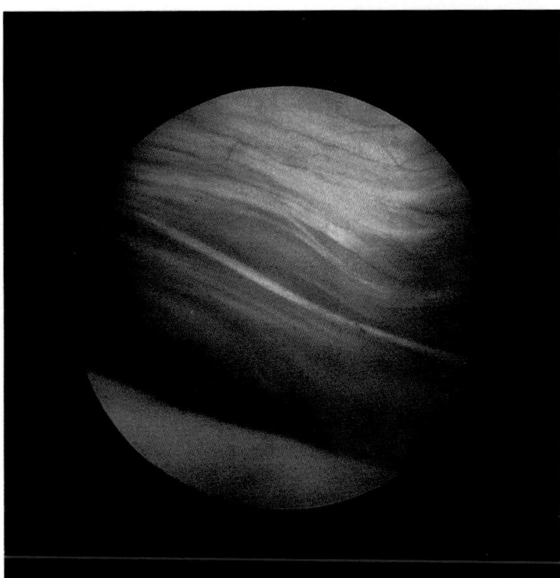

Figure 5.40
The undersurface of the acromion is covered by the insertion of the coracoacromial ligament.

flick from side to side (in fact it is the trochar flicking over the lateral edge of the ligament). If this manoeuvre is not performed, then the bursa may not be entered. If the arthroscope is not in the bursa when the fluid is switched on, it will create an extrabursal mass, which makes entry of the bursa almost impossible. The arthroscopist will then see an appearance as though the space was full of 'cobwebs' (Figure 5.37). If the bursa has been successfully entered, the arthroscopist will see a large synovially lined space (Figure 5.38). Orientation within this space is far more difficult than within the shoulder joint, and the insertion of two needles to mark the anterior edge of the acromion (Figure 5.39) – one at the lateral margin and another at the acromioclavicular joint – will help at this stage. The arthroscope is rotated upwards to examine the inferior surface of the acromion, which at this point is

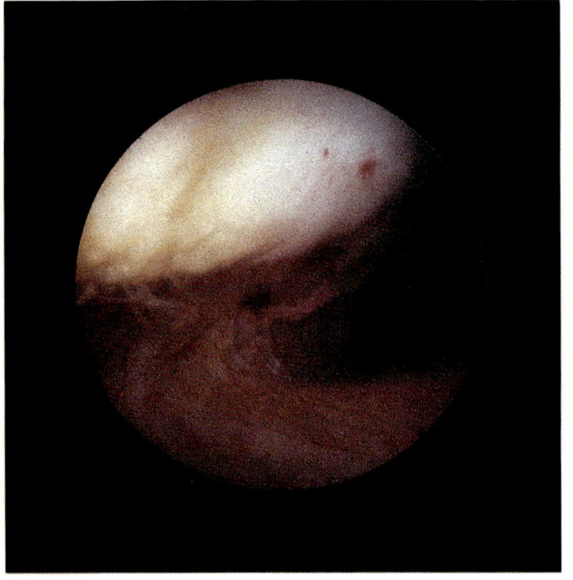

Figure 5.41

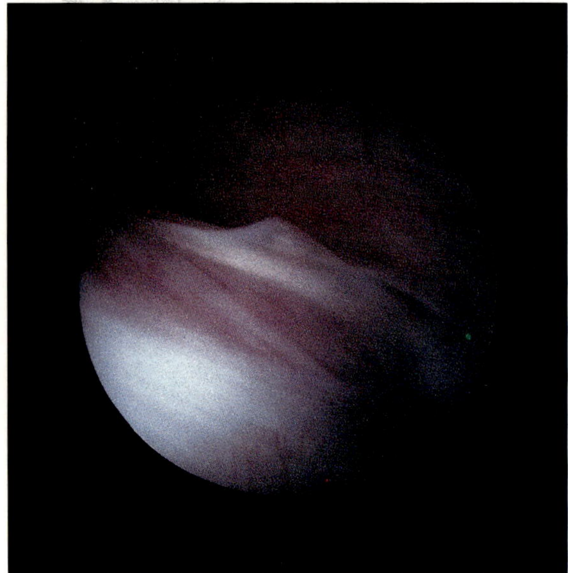

Figure 5.42

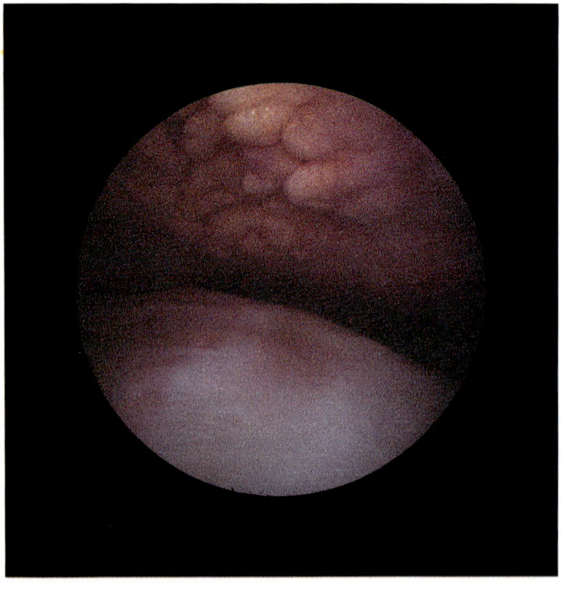

Figures 5.41, 5.42 and 5.43

The upper surface of the rotator cuff as seen during bursal endoscopy.

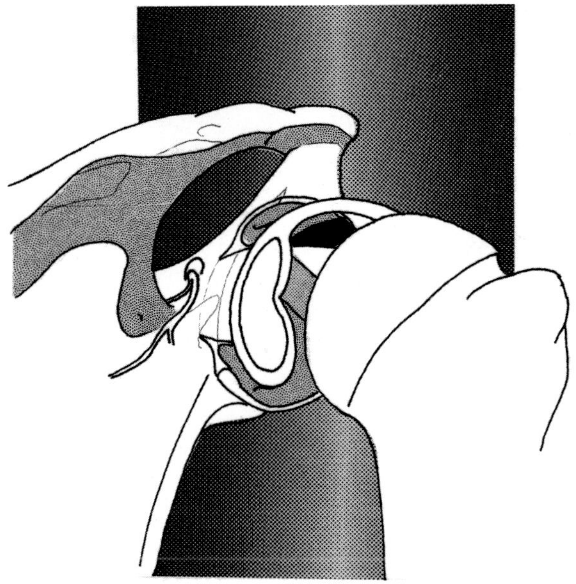

Figure 5.44
A simple pattern upon which the findings of shoulder arthroscopy can be drawn.

covered by the insertion of the coracoacromial ligament (Figure 5.40). Turning the arthroscope laterally, the edge of the acromion can be seen and the origin of the lateral multipennate section of the deltoid. The arthroscope is then rotated down to examine the superior surface of the rotator cuff (Figures 5.41, 5.42 and 5.43). When the examination is complete, the bursa is flushed out and the arthroscope and needles withdrawn. The skin puncture can be closed either with a single suture or with adhesive skin closure strips.

It is very important to make a drawing of the findings in the notes, as this is a far better reminder of what the joint and bursa actually looked like than a written documentary. A simple pattern upon which findings can be drawn is shown in Figure 5.44.

6 Abnormal findings

This chapter deals with the variety of abnormalities which can be seen arthroscopically, using the routine laid down in Chapter 5.

Long head of biceps

Fortunately, since the long head of biceps is the primary reference point of shoulder arthroscopy, abnormalities are seen in only some 10 per cent of cases. In patients with impingement, there may be fraying or tendinitis (Figure 6.1), often associated with changes in the rotator cuff. Some patients who have partial or full thickness rotator cuff tears may have debris hanging down into the joint obliterating the view of the long head of biceps (Figure 6.2). In some patients, the tendon may be missing following rupture. In approximately 3 per cent of patients, the long head of biceps will have a synovial mesentery, either complete (Figure 6.3), or represented by a strand (Figure 6.4), which should be considered as a variant of the norm.

Rotator cuff

A spectrum of abnormal changes can be found in the rotator cuff. The first evidence of impingement may be reddening of the cuff, and an increase in small-size vessels in the synovium (Figure 6.5). The next stage in the sequence is a 'hairy' degeneration of the cuff in the impingement area (close to the biceps tunnel) (Figure 6.6). The next stage is seen as a deep surface tear (Figure 6.7).

Finally, the partial thickness tear will give way to a full thickness tear (Figure 6.8), which matures to give rounded-off edges (Figure 6.9) through which can be seen bursal proliferation and the undersurface of the acromion (Figure 6.10).

Massive rotator cuff tears may be confusing initially. Instead of the rotator cuff the undersurface of the acromion is seen, and when probed it can be appreciated just how massive a cavity is present (Figures 6.11 and 6.12).

The glenoid labrum, inferior glenohumeral ligament complex

In traumatic dislocation, the labrum avulses from the glenoid rim (see pages 143–158), known as the Bankart lesion. This may give a variety of appearances. The normal labrum looks very similar to the meniscus of the knee (Figure 6.13). The usual pattern of the Bankart lesion is separation of the labrum from the rim (Figure 6.14), with a space visible both above

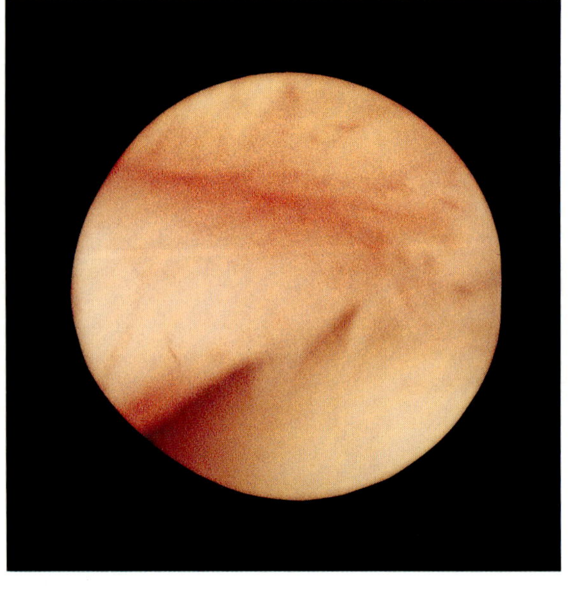

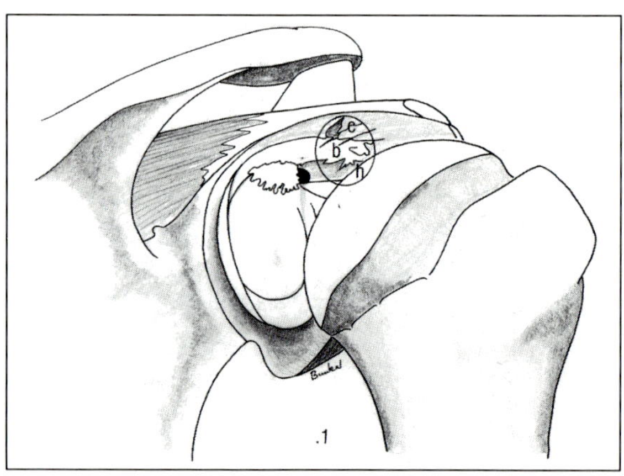

Figure 6.1

Fraying of the biceps tendon can be seen at the impingement point. c = cuff, b = biceps, h = humeral head.

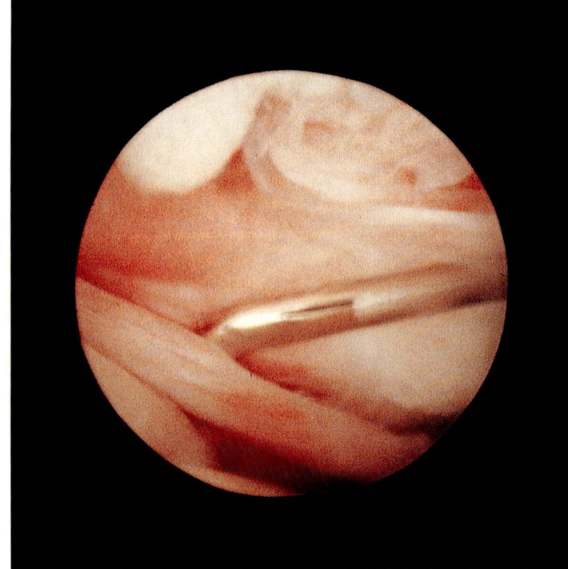

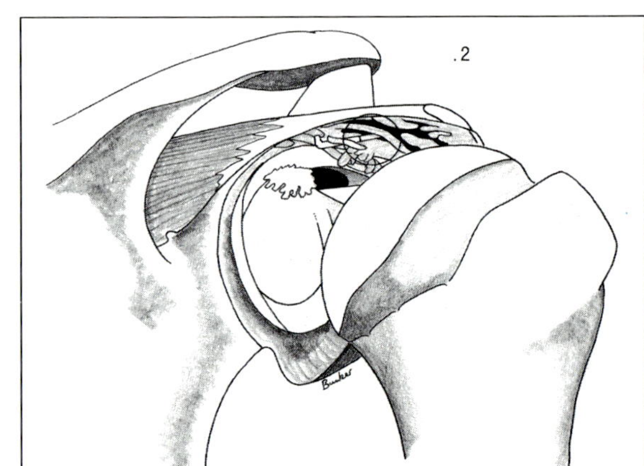

Figure 6.2

Sometimes the biceps tendon cannot be seen if tags from a rotator cuff tear hang down and hide it.

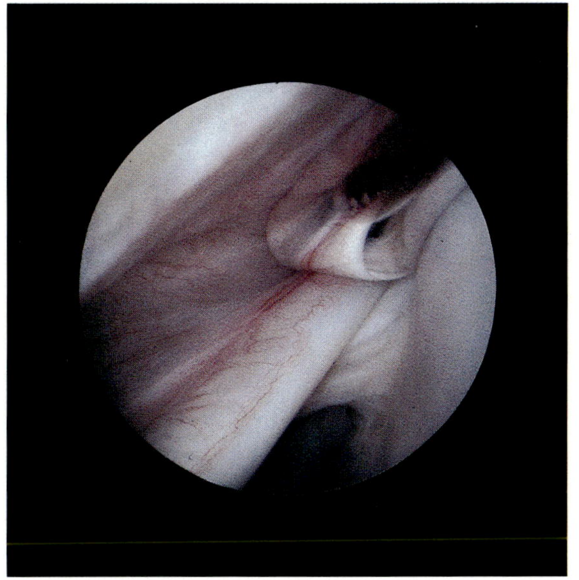

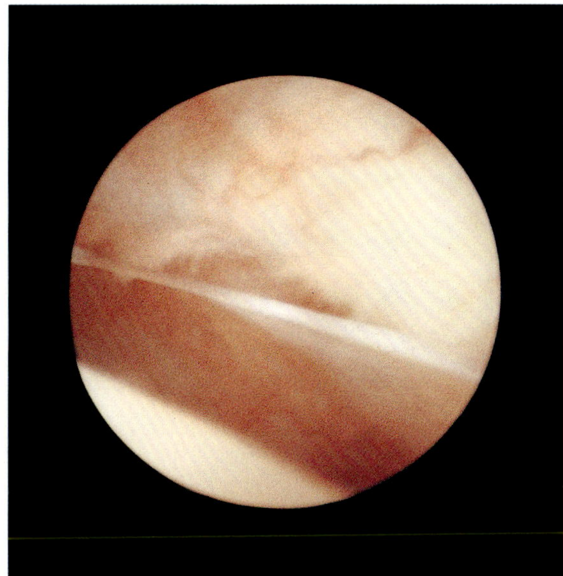

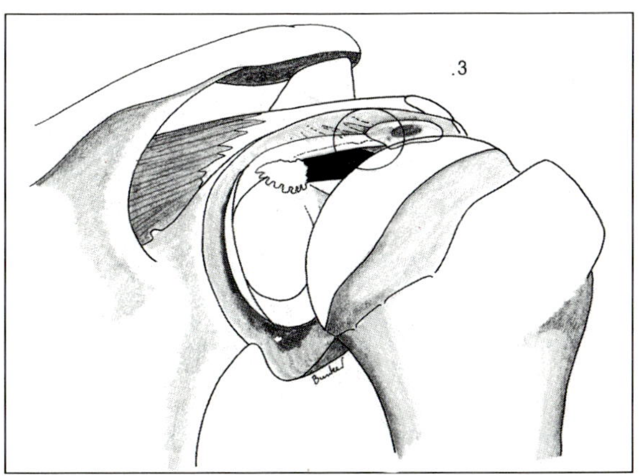

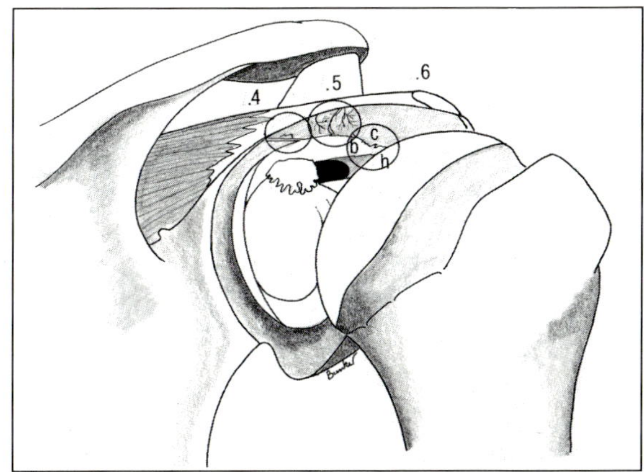

Figure 6.3

The biceps tendon may be enfolded by a mesentery. This is not an abnormal finding but a variation of normal.

Figure 6.4

The mesentery to biceps tendon may be represented by a single strand which could be taken for an adhesion.

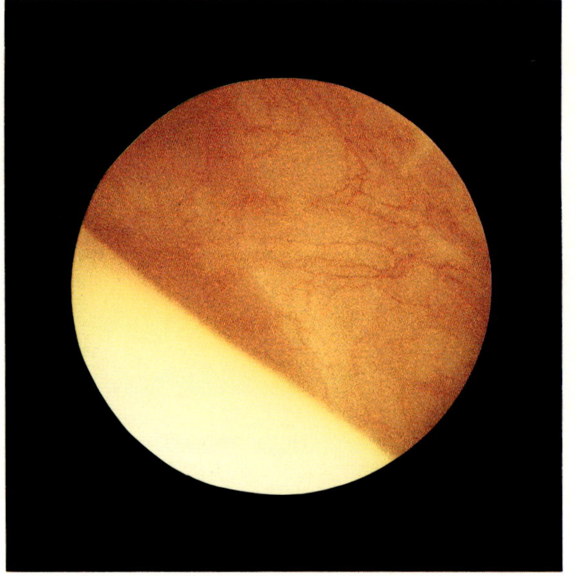

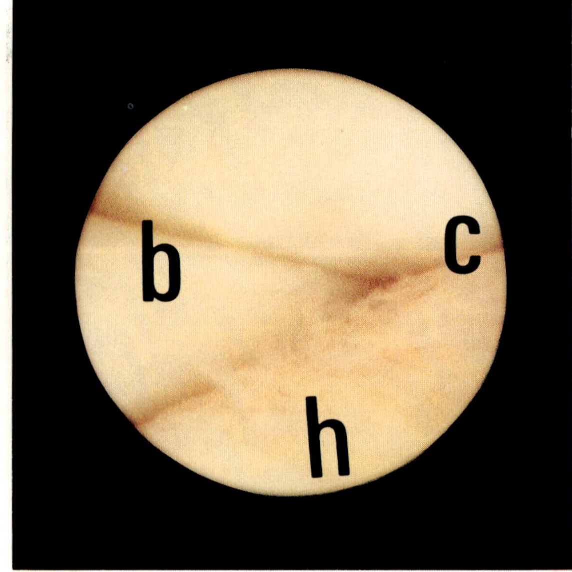

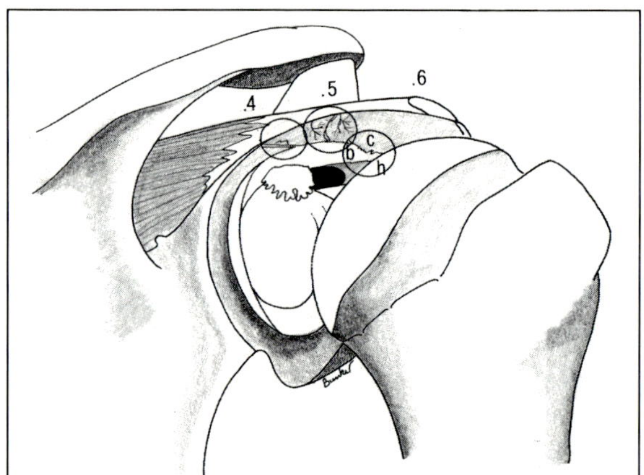

Figure 6.5

Vasculitis of the rotator cuff.

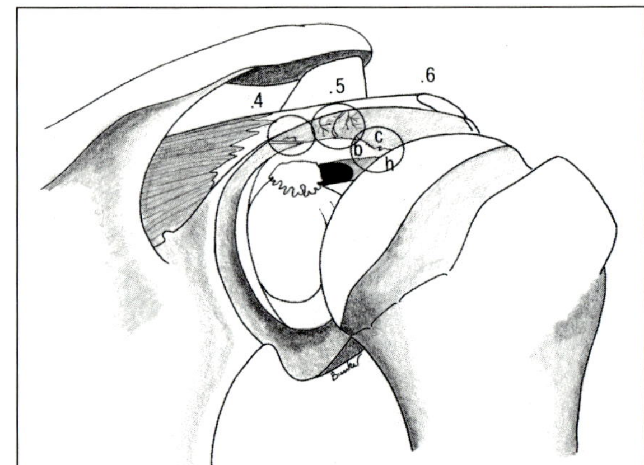

Figure 6.6

Fraying of the rotator cuff at the impingement point. c = cuff, b = biceps, h = humeral head.

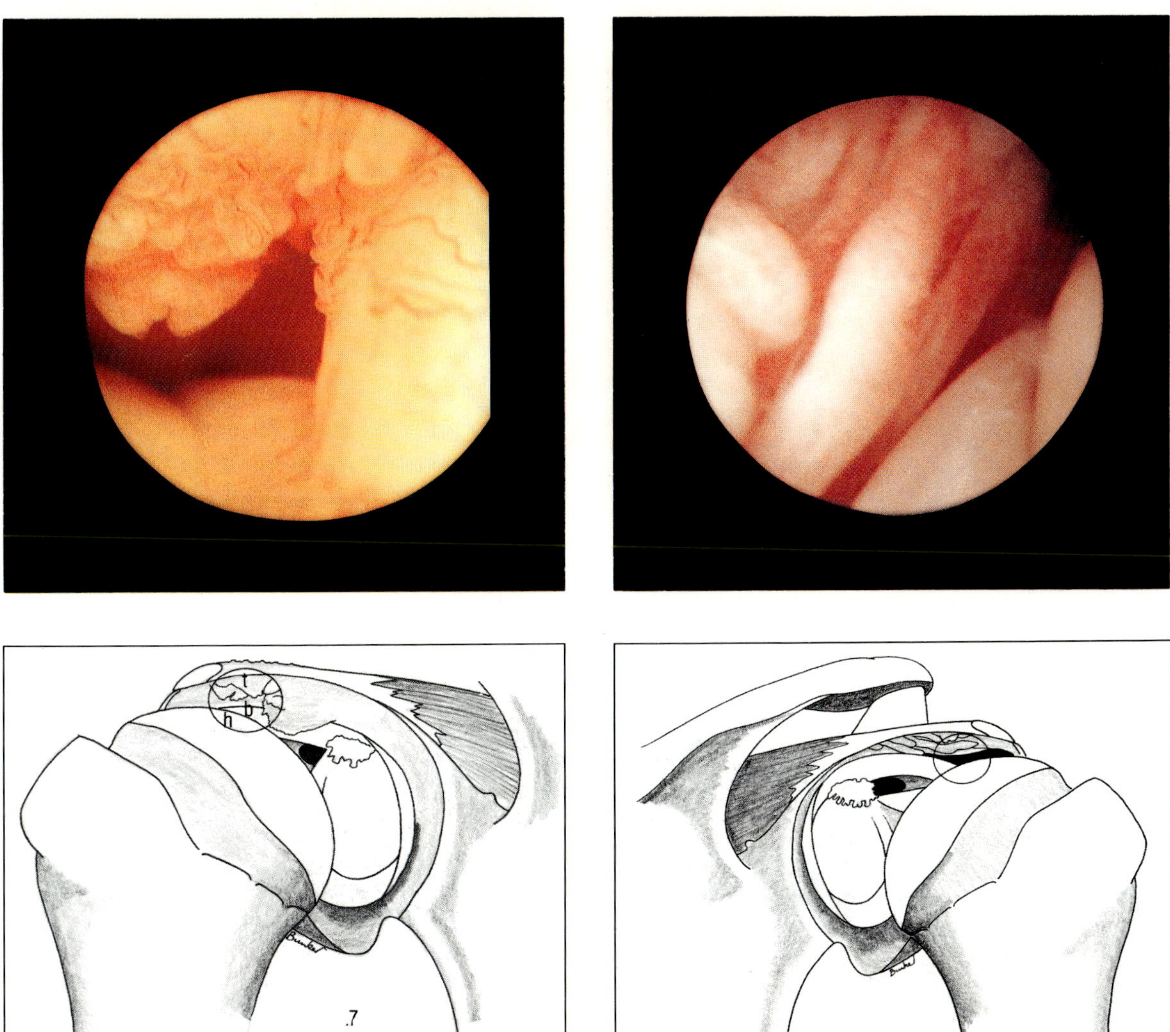

Figure 6.7

Partial thickness rotator cuff tear covered with thickened synovium.

Figure 6.8

Full thickness rotator cuff tear.

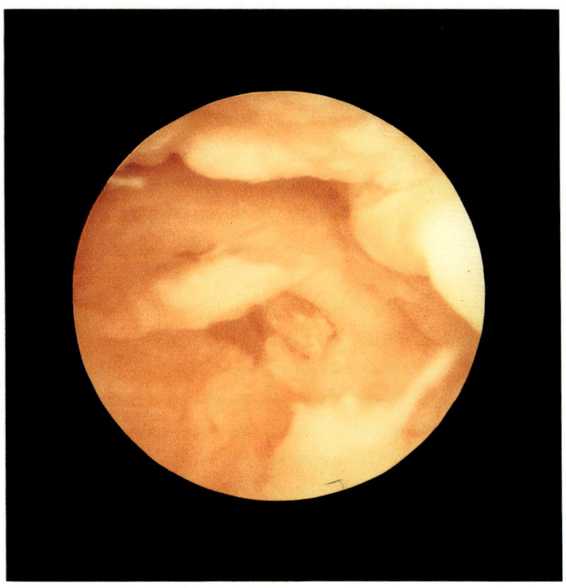

Figure 6.9

A full thickness rotator cuff tear has rounded mature edges and the proliferative bursal tissue hangs down through it.

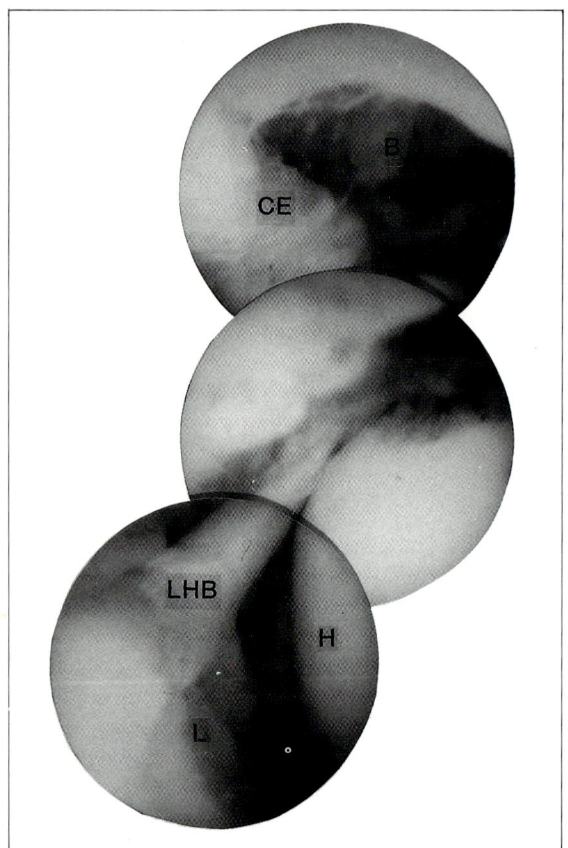

Figure 6.10

A collage of arthroscopic photographs to show the rotator cuff tear seen in Figure 6.9 in relation to the rest of the joint.

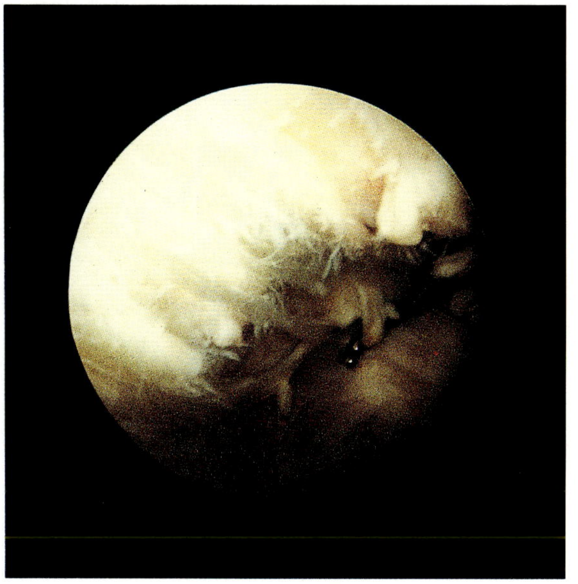

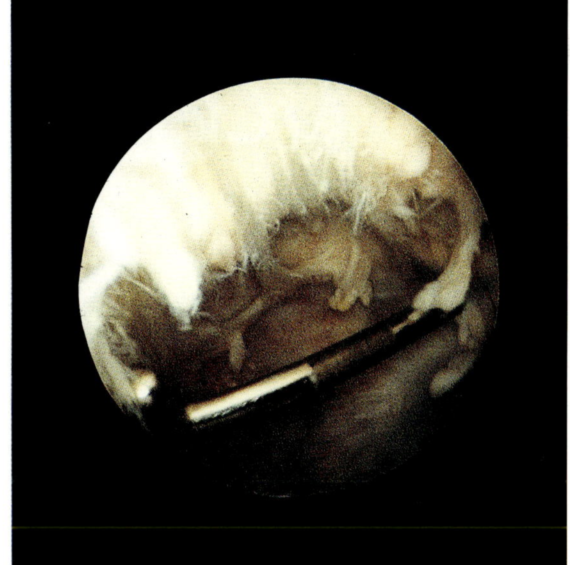

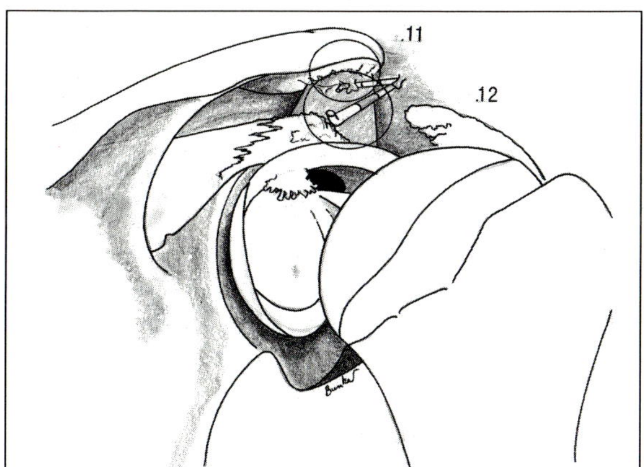

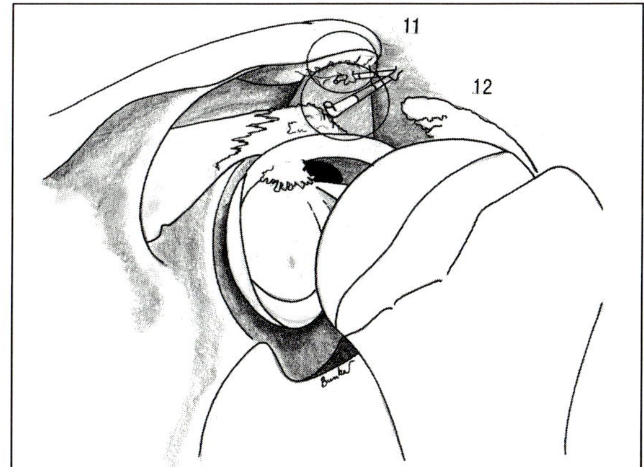

Figures 6.11 and 6.12

In a massive rotator cuff tear, the edges may not be seen. There is just a large and very irregular cavity, the size of which can be judged by the extent to which the hook probe travels.

Figure 6.12

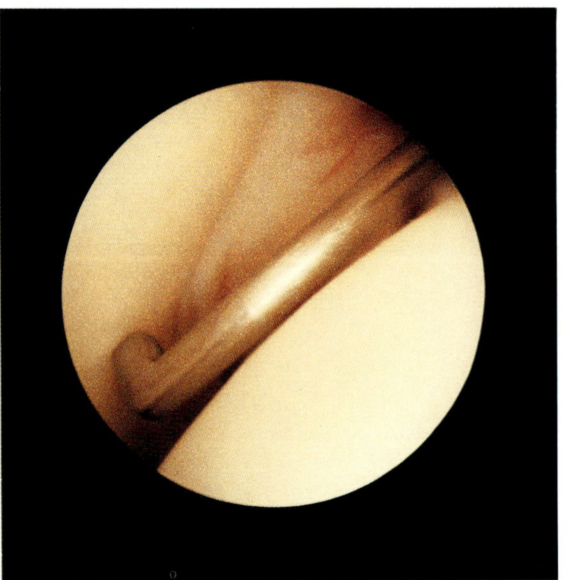

Figure 6.13

The normal labrum looks similar in appearance to the normal knee meniscus.

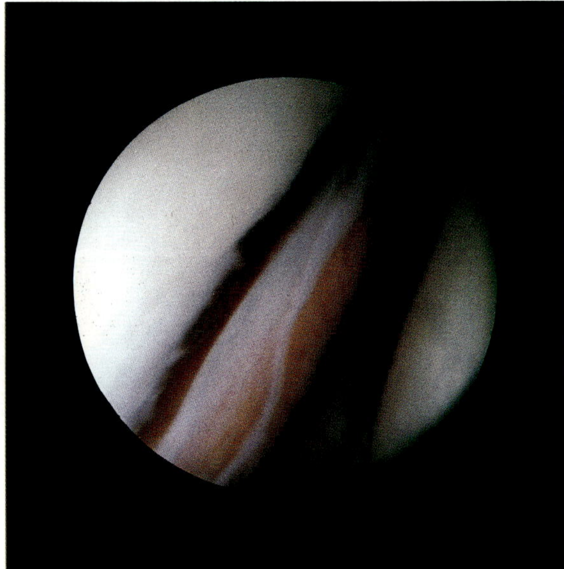

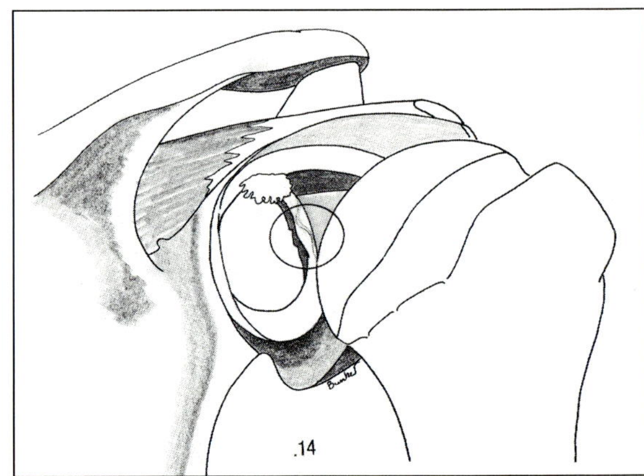

Figure 6.14

The usual Bankart appearance of separation between the glenoid and the labrum.

and below the labrum. Another appearance is where the avulsed labrum prolapses over the front of the glenoid (Figure 6.15). Finally, if there has been a high number of episodes of dislocation then the labrum and the associated glenohumeral ligaments will be torn, shredded and eventually disappear (Figure 6.16). The anterior rim of the glenoid will become crevassed by repeated episodes of dislocation (Figures 6.17 and 6.18).

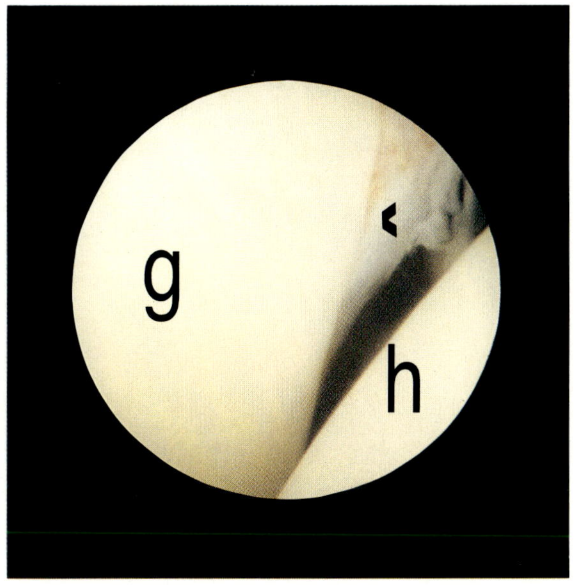

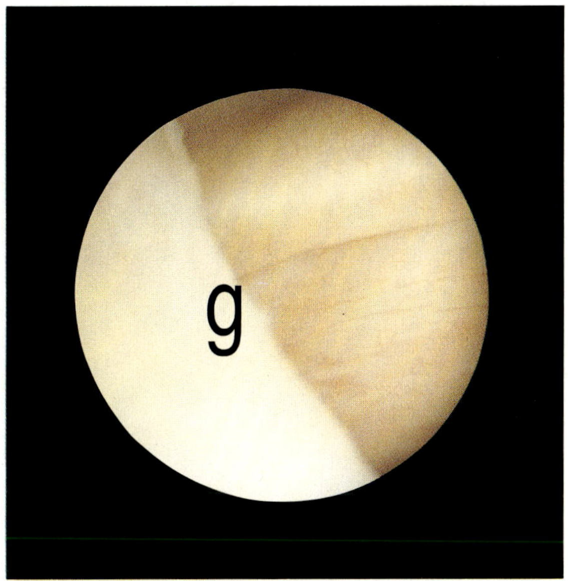

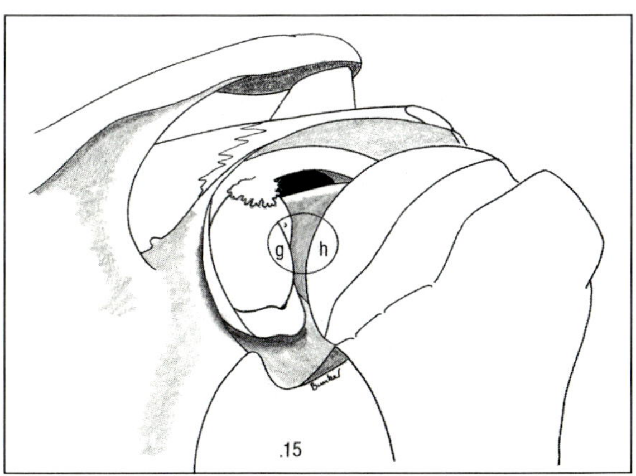

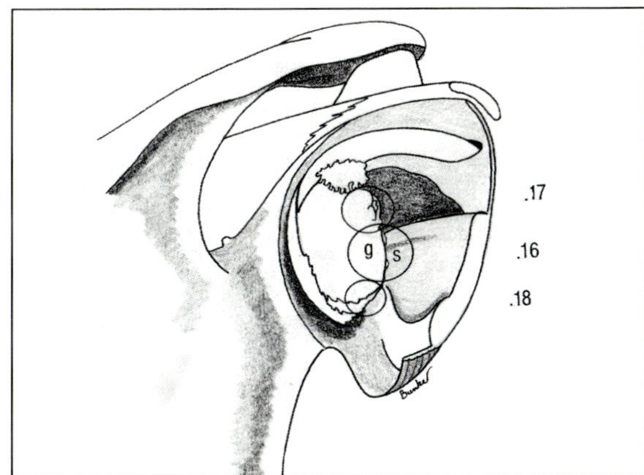

Figure 6.15

The labrum may prolapse in front of the glenoid rim in the 'over-the-top' type of Bankart lesion.

Figure 6.16

After several episodes of dislocation, the labrum becomes disrupted. Along with the middle glenohumeral ligament, it may eventually disappear altogether, g = glenoid, s = subscapularis tendon.

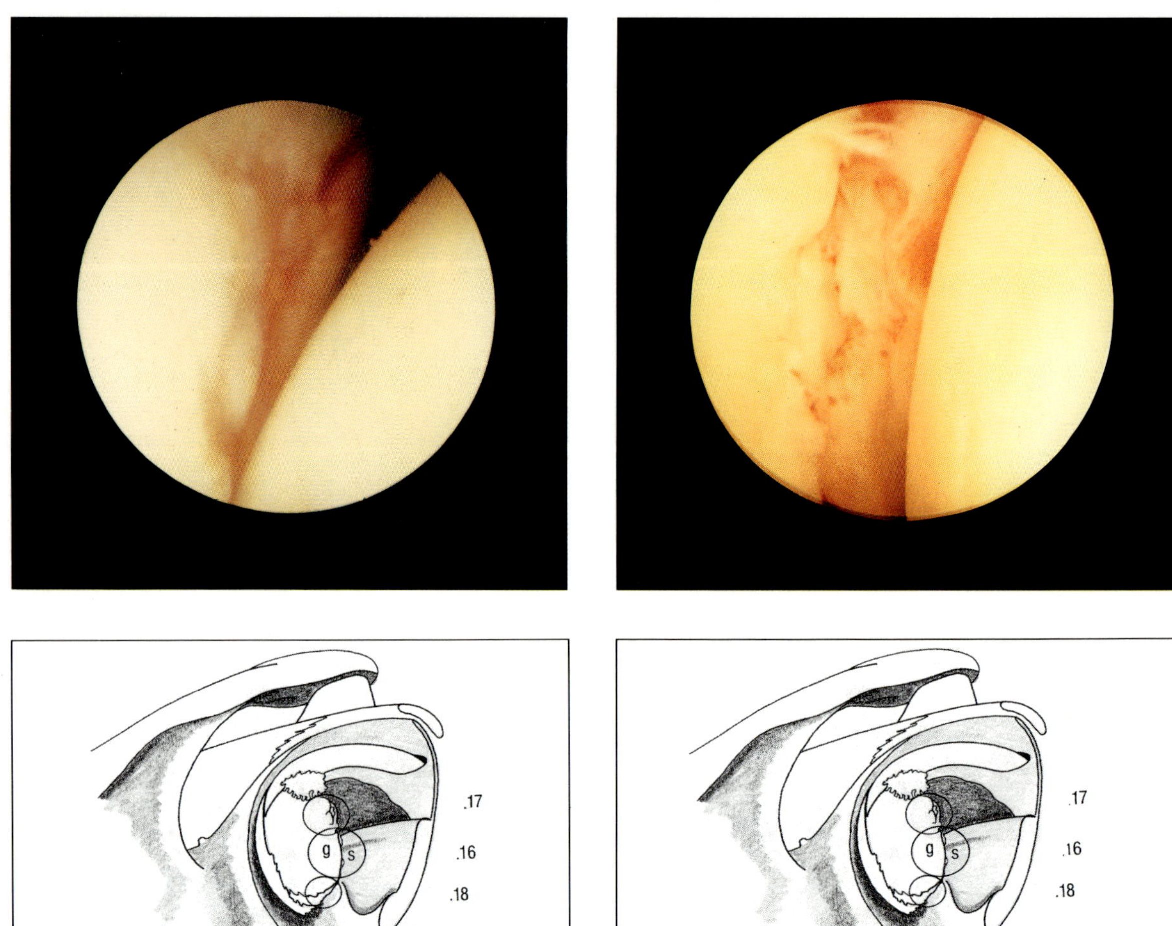

Figures 6.17 and 6.18

The front edge of the glenoid may become crevassed.

Figure 6.18

Labral tears

If the labrum is torn or avulsed in the inferior two-thirds of its extent, this usually signifies a Bankart lesion. However, there is some discussion about tears in the upper third (Figures 6.19 and 6.20), and tears without separation.

Detrisac[1] has described a normal separation of the labrum in the upper third, occurring in some 80 per cent of the cadavers he examined. Others have described a superior tear, or avulsion of the superior labrum and the origin of the long head of biceps, which may be common in throwing sports. This is thought to be caused by the pull of biceps in the deceleration phase of elbow extension.

Glenohumeral ligaments

The normal appearance of the glenohumeral ligaments on pages 85–93 has been discussed (see also Figure 6.21). The middle glenohumeral ligament is variable, from a thin translucent sheet to a strong thick ligament. It may be absent following repeated dislocation (see Chapter 9 and Figure 6.22). The inferior glenohumeral ligament should be considered as a prolongation of the anterior labrum (Figure 6.23).

Inferior glenohumeral recess

In the normal shoulder the inferior glenohumeral recess is a large cavity (see Figure 5.27). The recess may be constricted in patients with a stiff painful shoulder (frozen shoulder). The inferior glenohumeral recess is a favourite hiding place for loose bodies, which vary in size from a needle point (Figure 6.24) to large bodies (Figures 6.25 and 6.26). The usual source of loose bodies is the Hill–Sachs impaction fracture of dislocation.

Posterior labrum

The posterior labrum may be torn, just as the anterior labrum. However, this does not signify a posterior dislocation as anterior dislocation may cause a tear of the posterior labrum (see Chapter 9).

Hill–Sachs lesions

Once more, a spectrum of lesions can be seen on the back of the humeral head depending on the energy of the initial dislocation episode, and the frequency of dislocation. Hill–Sachs lesions can vary from a small cartilaginous dimple (Figure 6.27), to a full-blown osteochondral defect (Figures 6.28, 6.29, 6.30 and 6.31). It should be re-emphasized that the normal humeral head has a bare area of bone between the posterior synovial reflection and the cartilaginous surface (Figures 6.32 and 6.33), which must not be confused with a Hill–Sachs lesion.

Abnormalities of the synovium

Synovitis is common in patients with the so-called frozen shoulder syndrome (see Chapter 7). Wiley[2] describes a particular pattern of synovitis arising in the foramen of Weitbrecht which is very red and vascular.

Arthritis

Osteoarthritis is rare in the shoulder joint. The appearance of the cartilage of both the glenoid and the humerus parallels the pattern of the disease in other joints (Figures 6.35, 6.36 and 6.37).

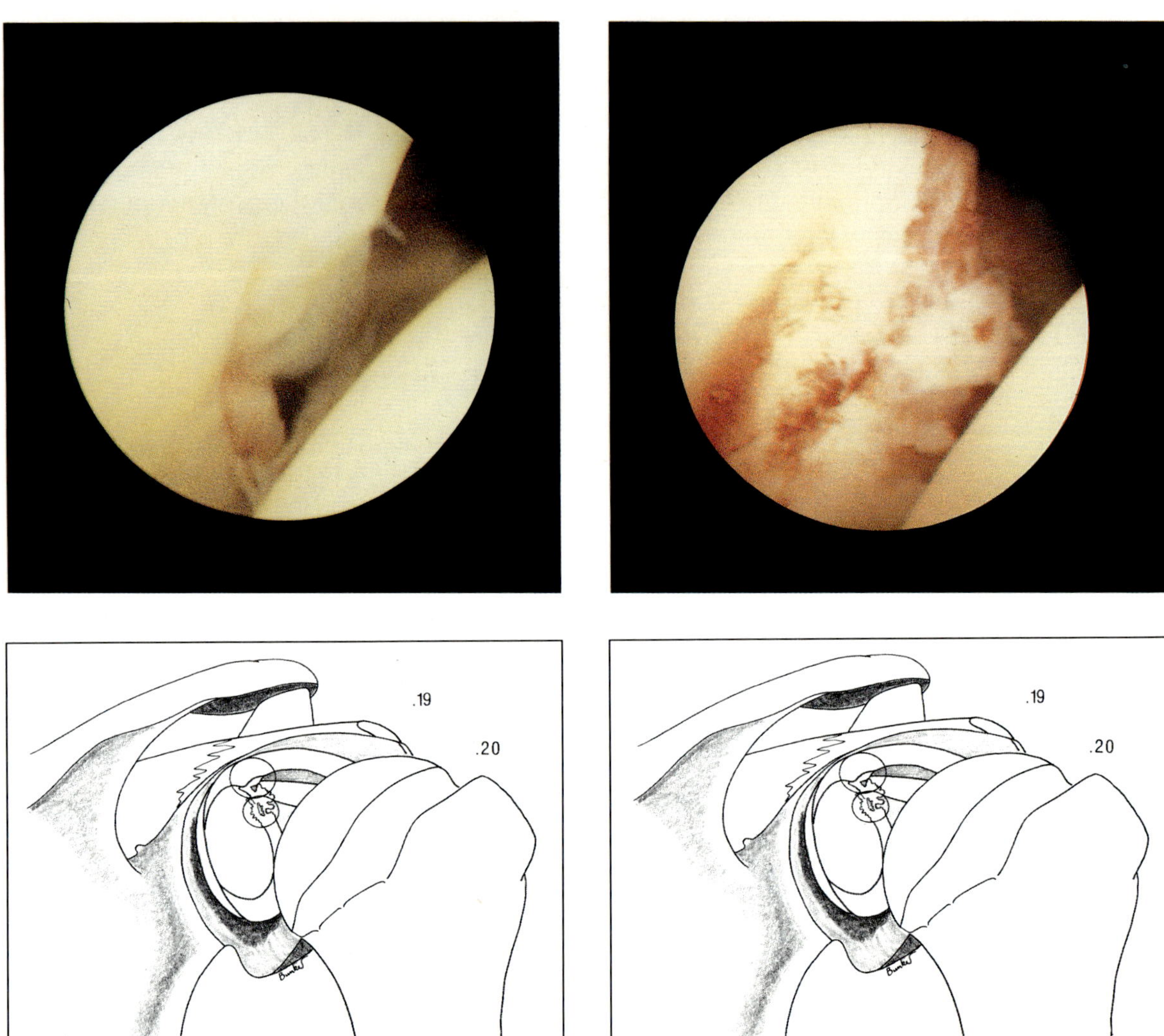

Figures 6.19 and 6.20

Tears of the glenoid labrum.

Figure 6.20

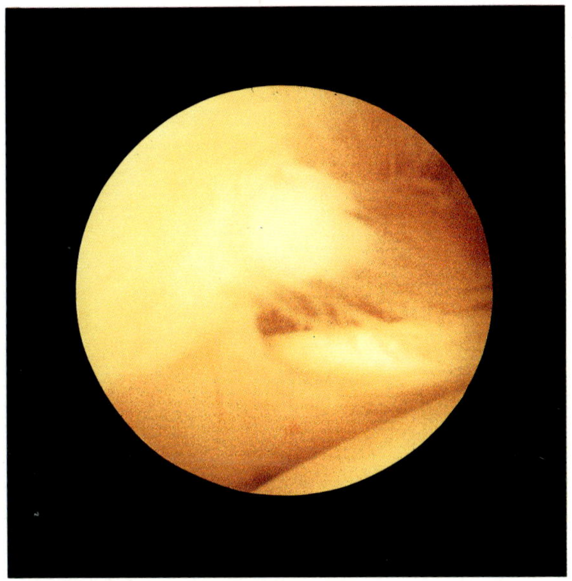

Figure 6.21
The normal middle glenohumeral ligament passing obliquely over the intra-articular upper edge of the subscapularis tendon.

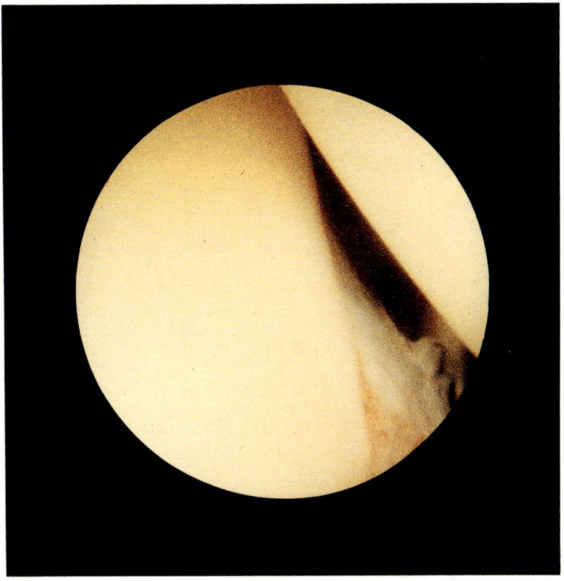

Figure 6.22
Absent middle glenohumeral ligament.

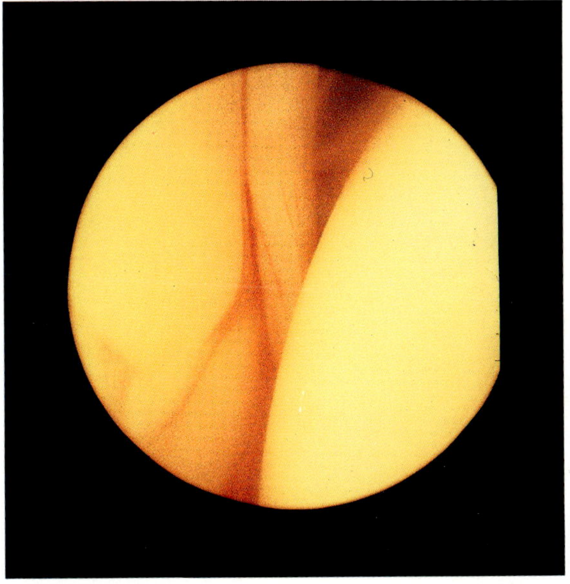

Figure 6.23
The inferior glenohumeral ligament as a prolongation of the labrum.

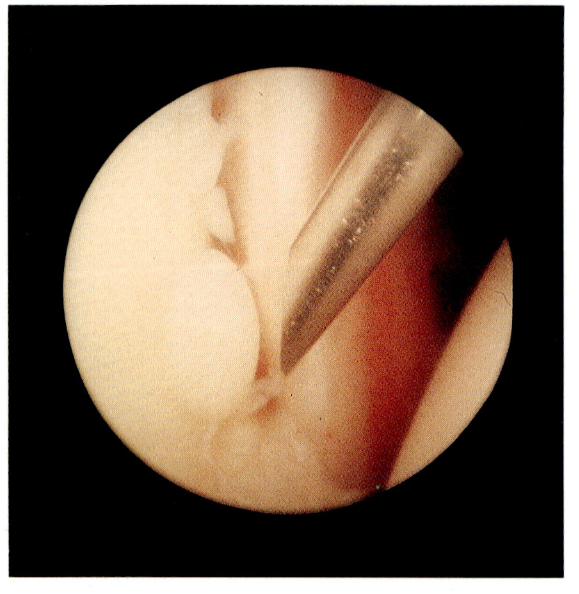

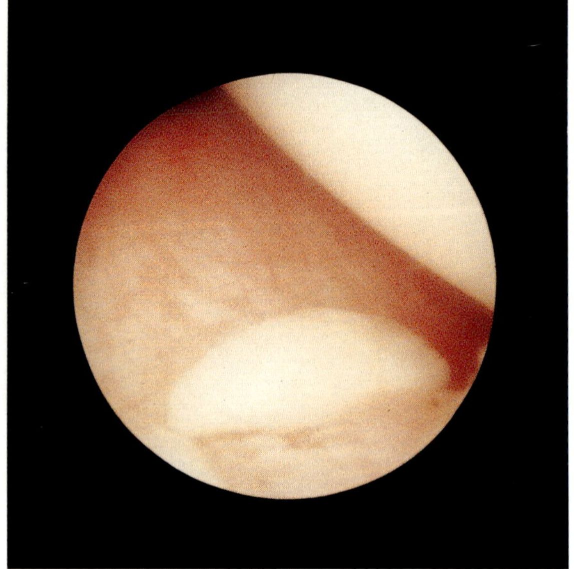

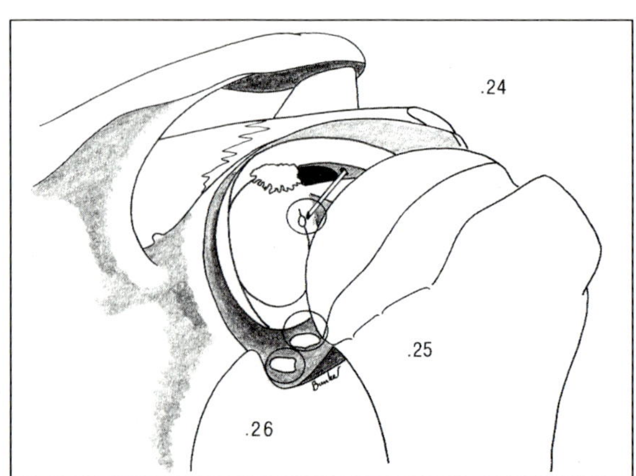

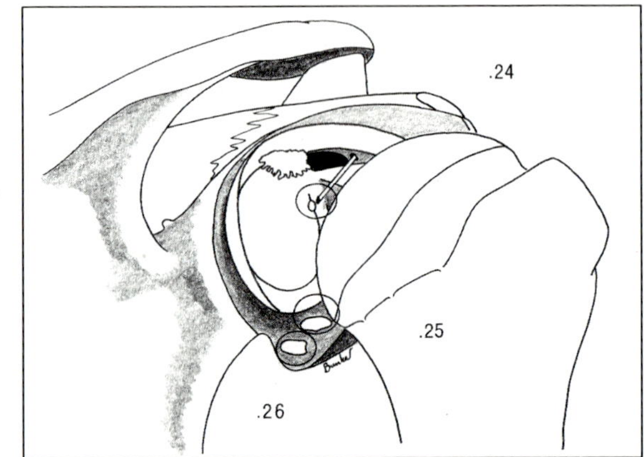

Figure 6.24

A small loose body the size of a needle.

Figures 6.25 and 6.26

Larger loose bodies.

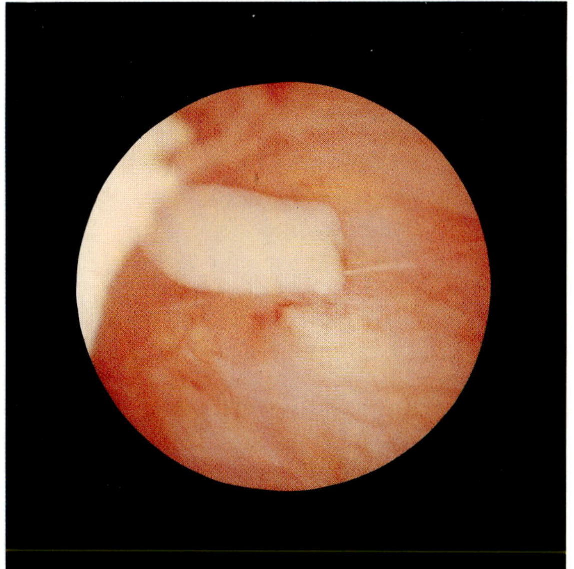

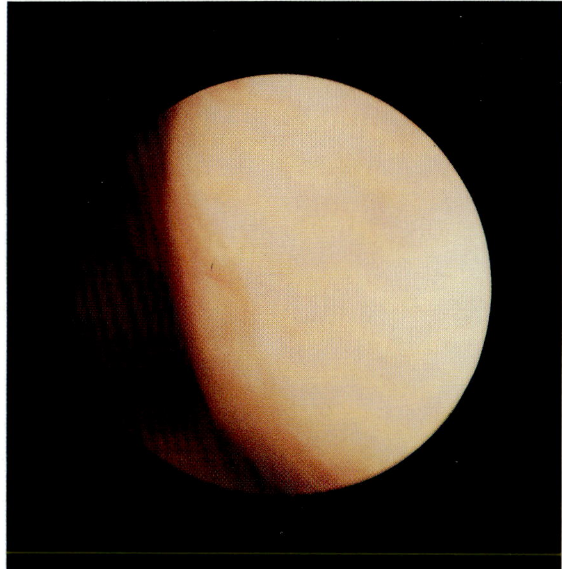

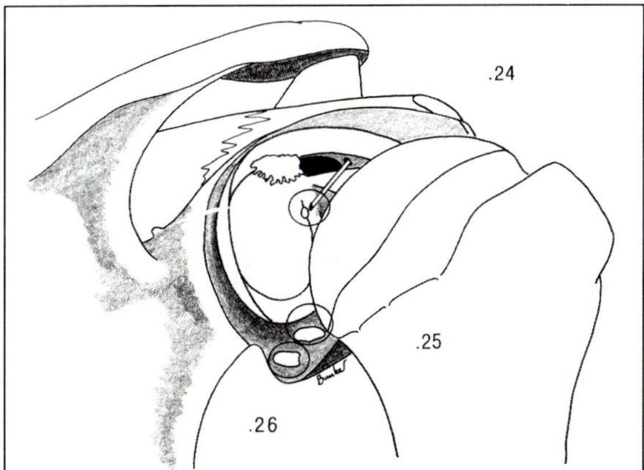

Figure 6.26

Figure 6.27

Hill–Sachs defect can be a small dimple.

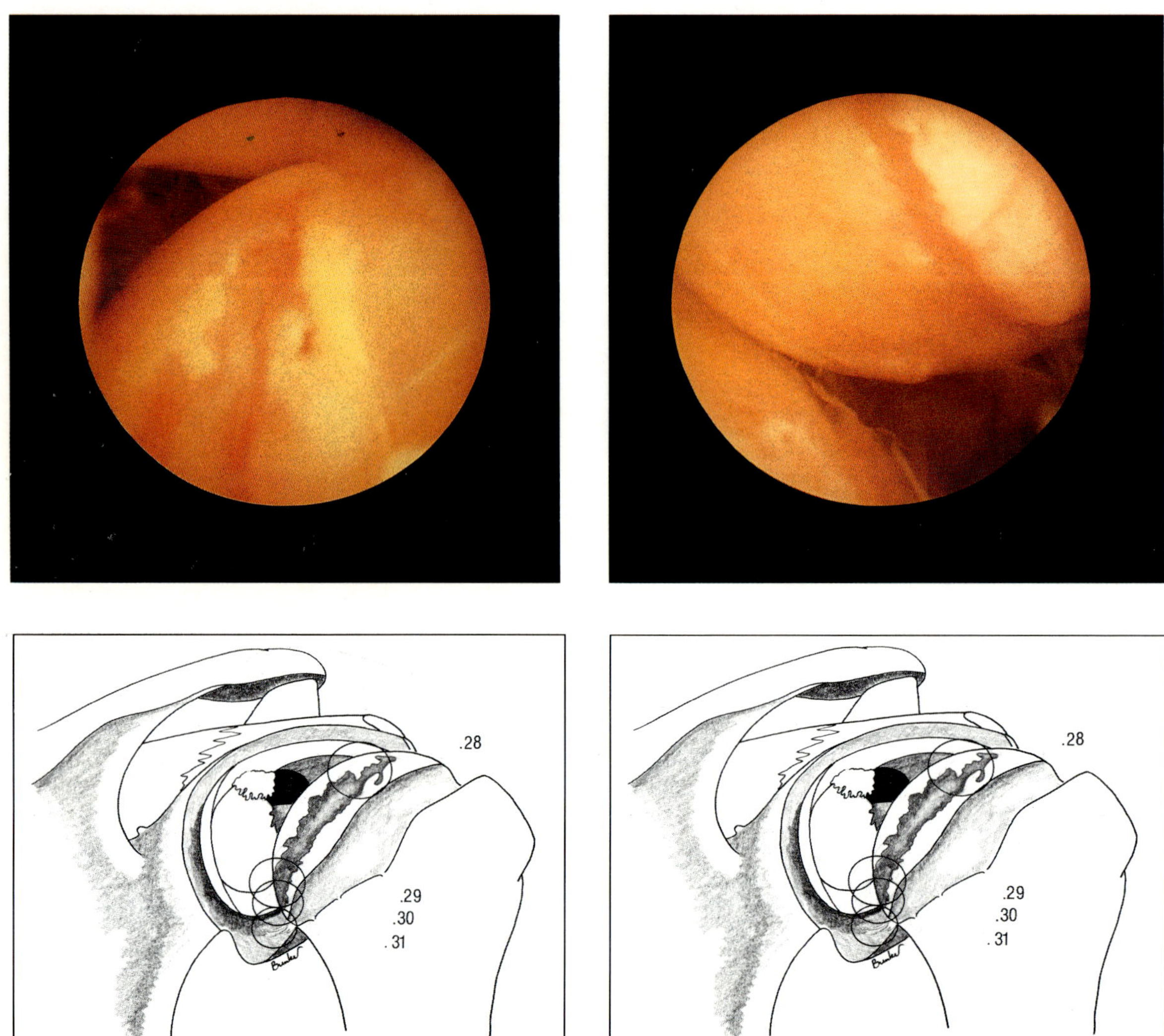

Figures 6.28, 6.29, 6.30 and 6.31
A large Hill–Sachs defect.

Figure 6.29

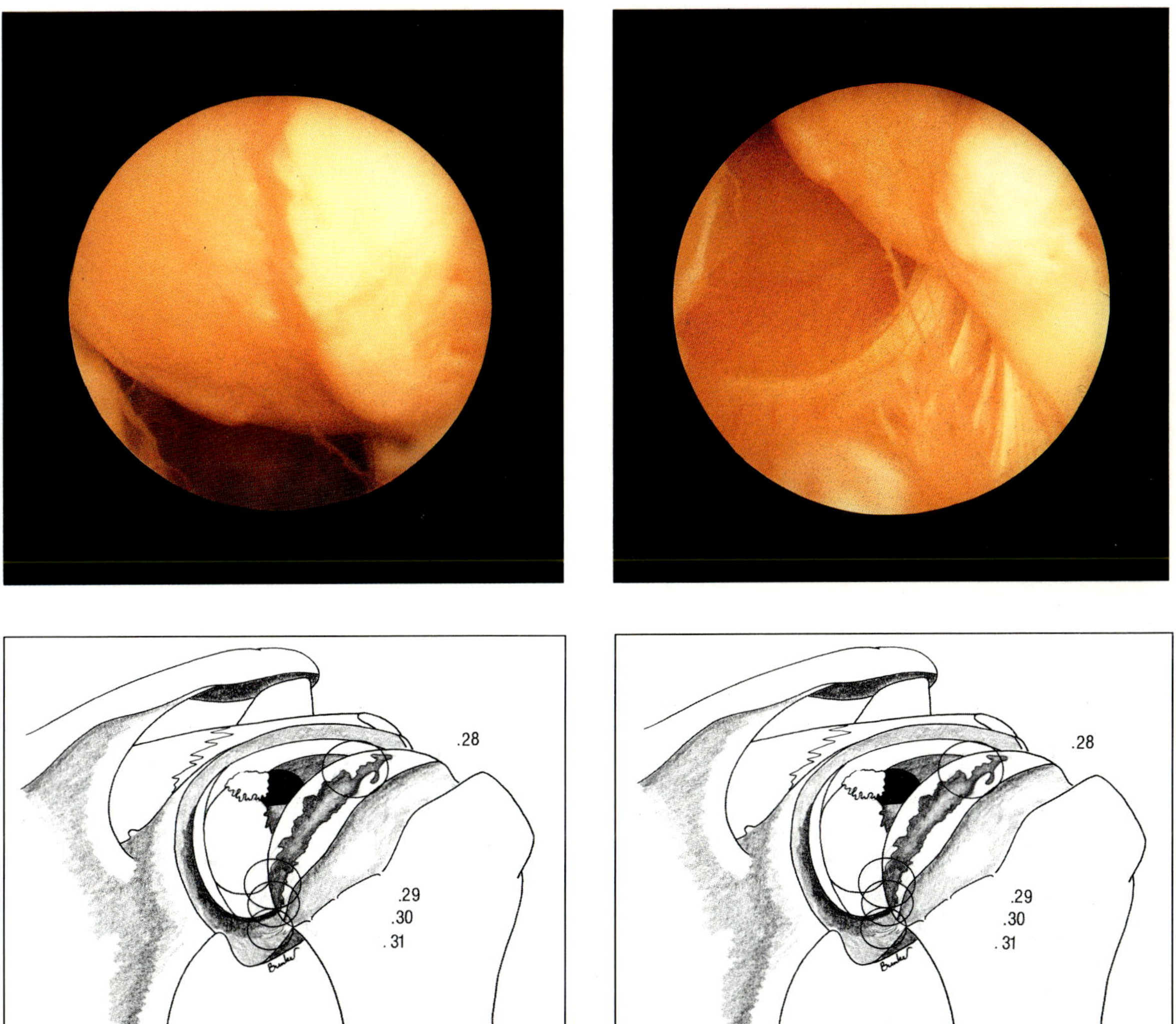

Figure 6.30

Figure 6.31

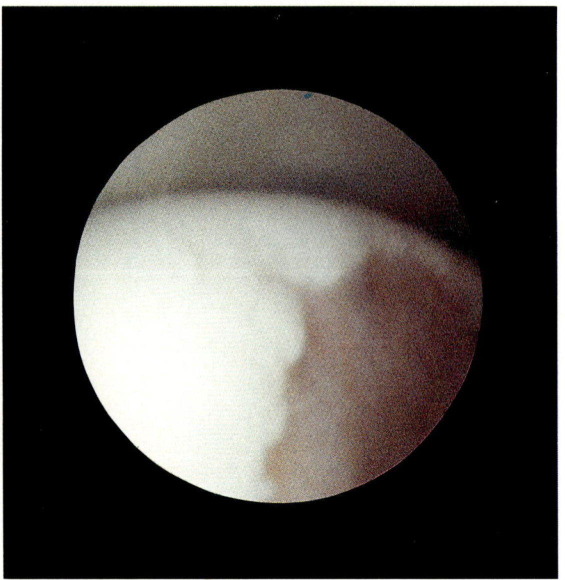

Figures 6.32 and 6.33

The bare area of the humeral head should not be mistaken for a Hill–Sachs defect. Note the difference from 6.28 to 6.31 in that there is no articular cartilage to the right (reflection side) of the bare area.

Figure 6.33

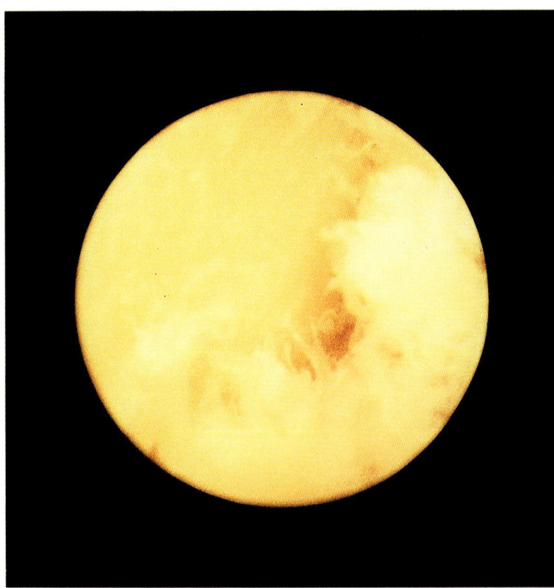

Figure 6.34

Crystal deposition on the synovium.

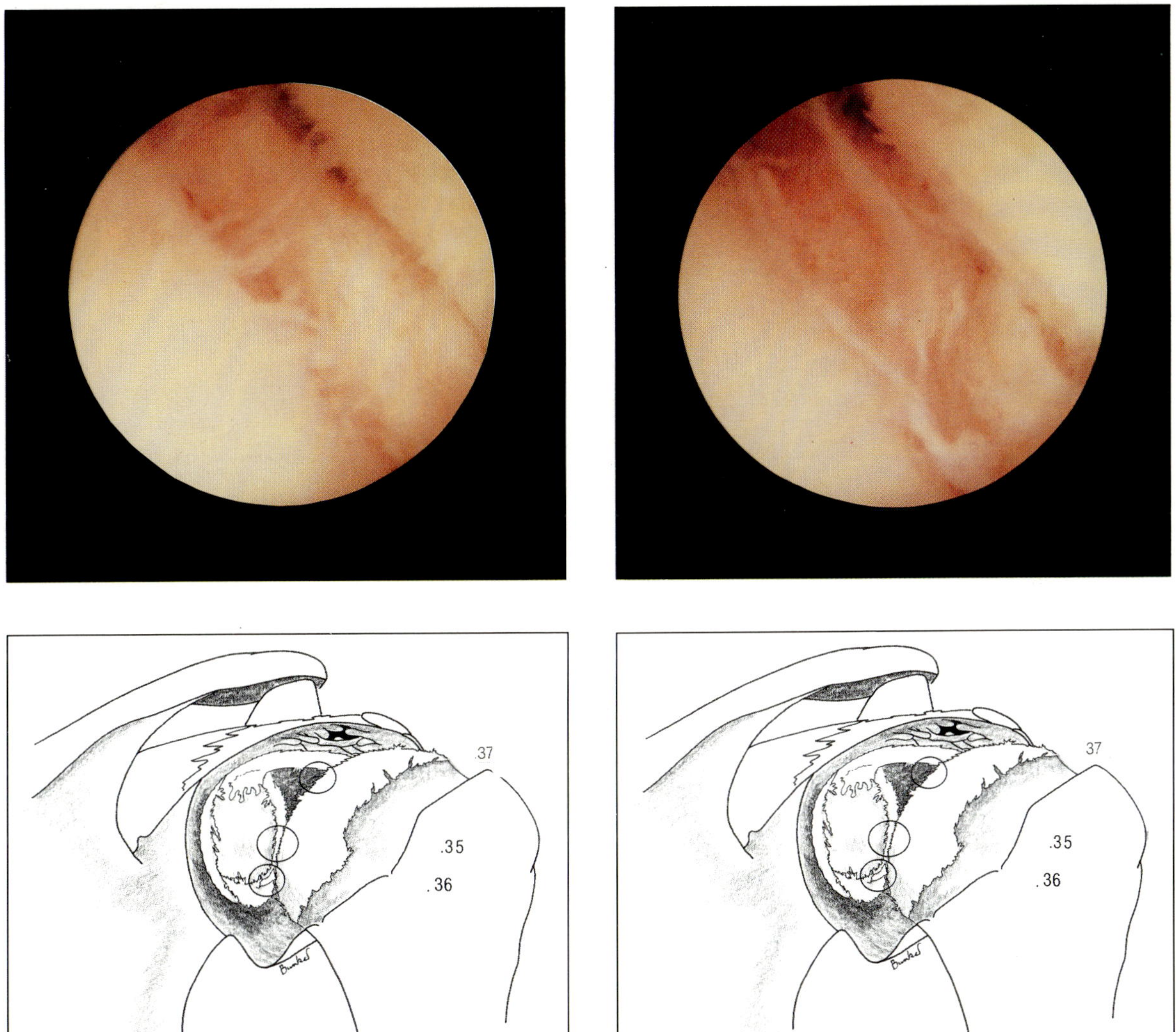

Figures 6.35, 6.36 and 6.37
Arthritic joint surfaces in the shoulder.

Figure 6.36

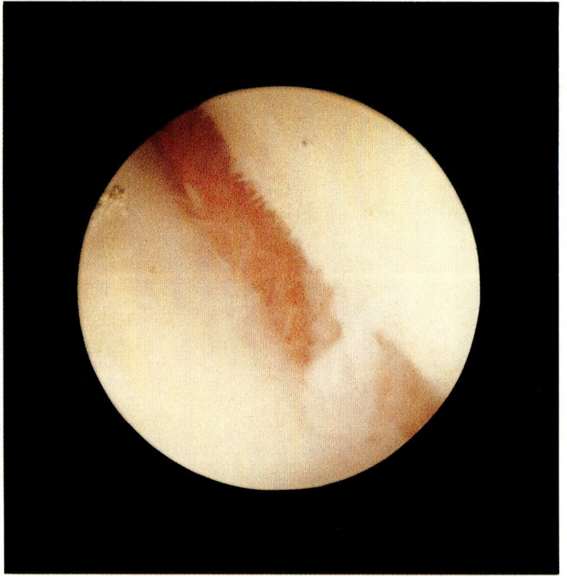

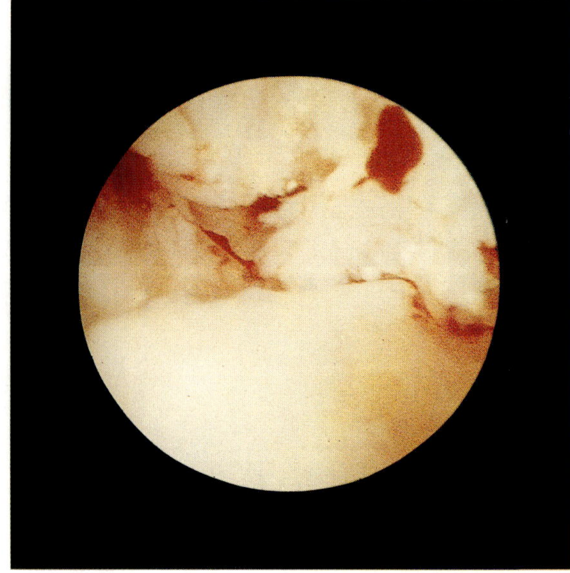

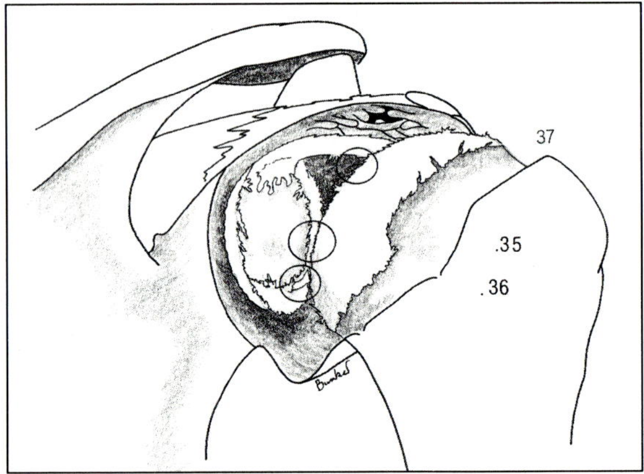

Figure 6.37

Figure 6.38

Vascular pannus eroding the articular surface of the humeral head.

Rheumatoid arthritis commonly affects the shoulder joint. In the early stages, there is an aggressive synovitis. Pannus can be seen eroding the cartilage in the humeral head (Figure 6.38).

Fractures

It is rare to arthroscope a patient with a glenoid fracture. The case with a displaced glenoid fracture shown in Figures 6.39 and 6.40 was

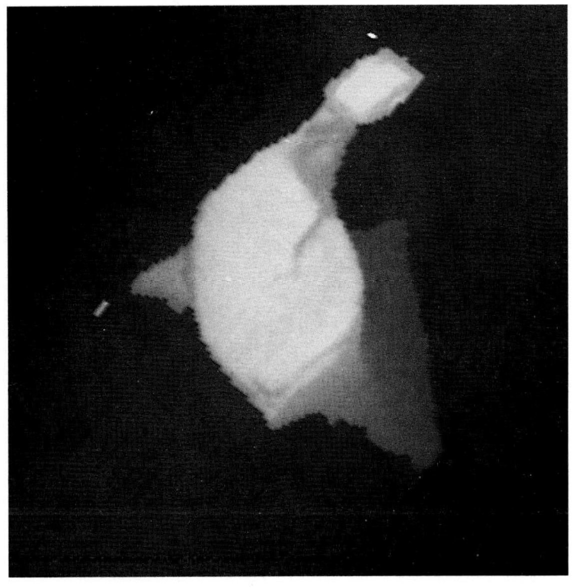

Figures 6.39 and 6.40

Three-dimensional subtraction CT scan of a fracture of the glenoid.

arthroscoped prior to open reduction and internal fixation to assess whether the maximum incongruity was at the front or back, in order to plan the approach as the three-dimensional computer tomography (3D CT) reconstruction program had temporarily gone down. Bleeding from fractures is more difficult to control in the shoulder than the knee, making the photography of poor quality (Figure 6.41), but the major incongruity could be seen anteriorly, and an anterior approach was used for reconstruction.

Joint replacement

Again it is extremely rare to arthroscope a patient following a shoulder replacement. One patient had residual pain following his second shoulder replacement, the eighth operation on this shoulder. He had a small radiolucent line

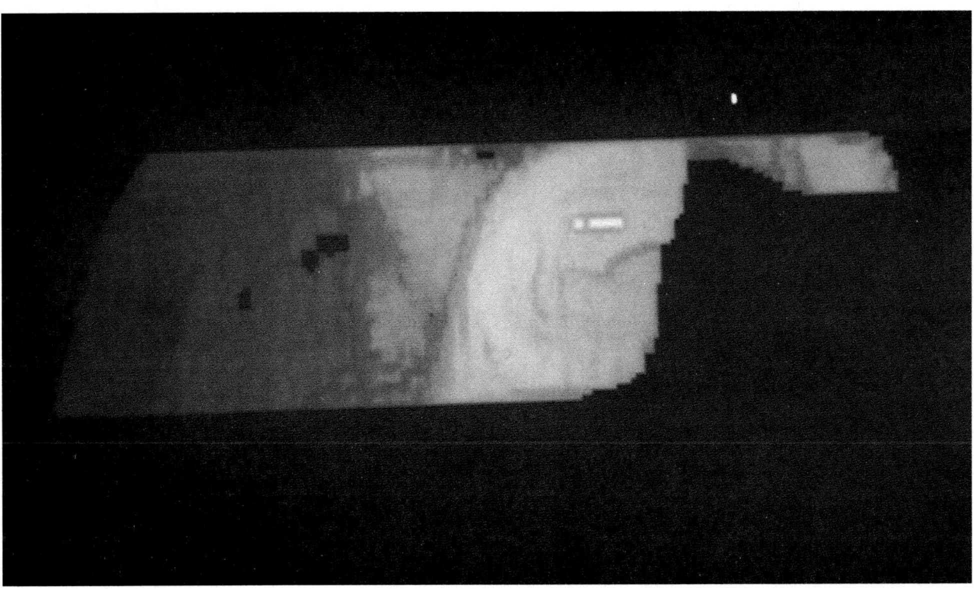

Figure 6.40

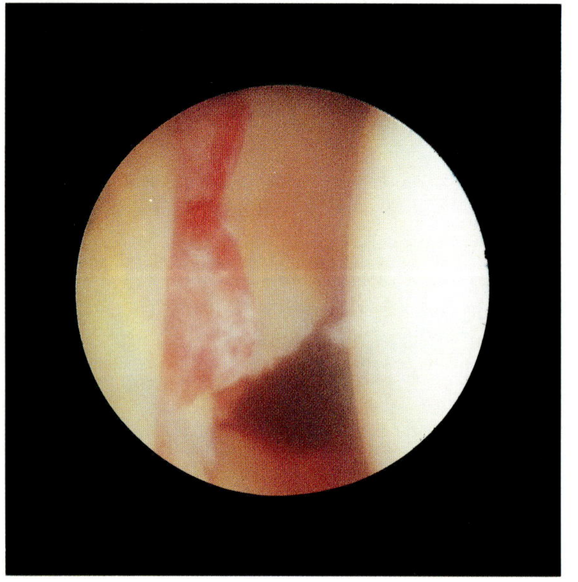

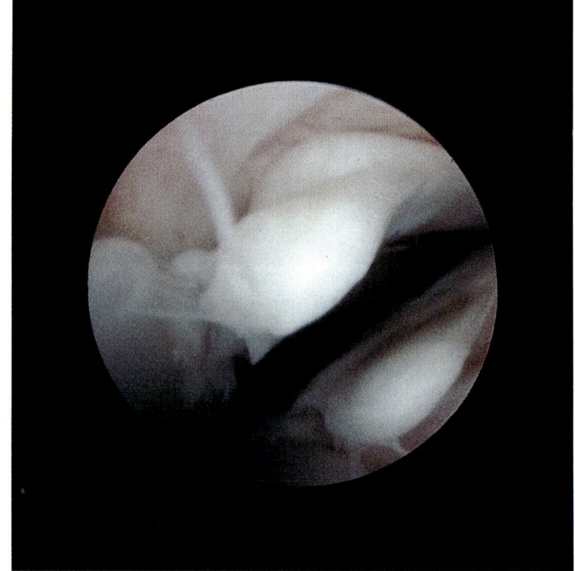

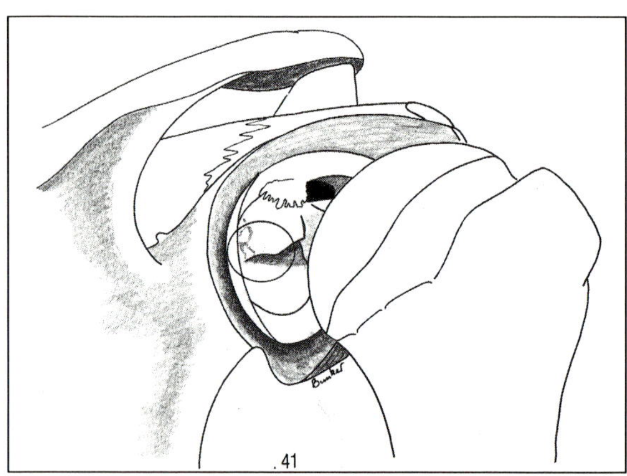

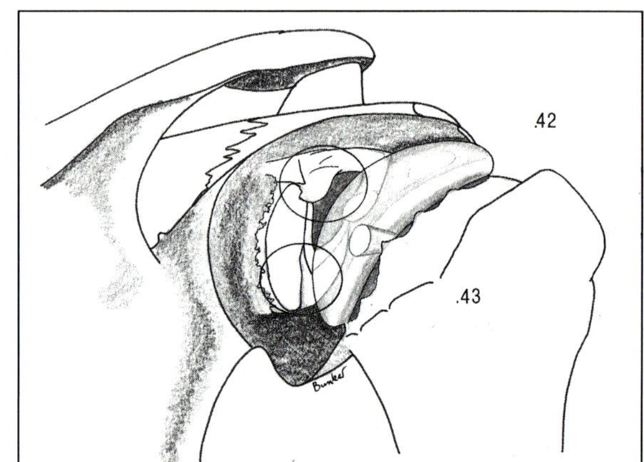

Figure 6.41

The fracture could be visualized arthroscopically, although the field was distorted due to bleeding.

Figures 6.42 and 6.43

Neer shoulder replacement visualized arthroscopically.

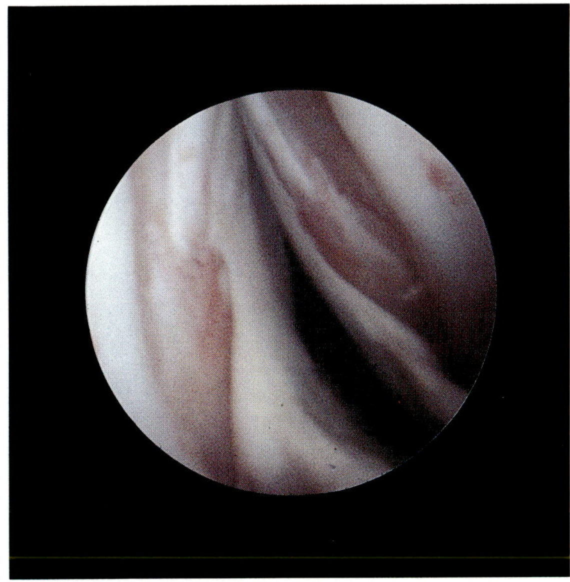

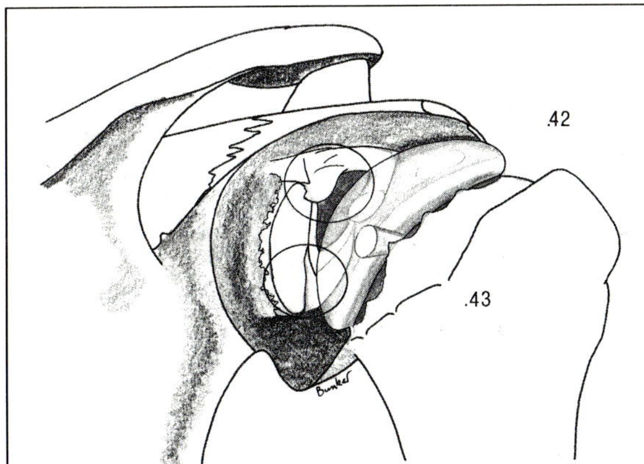

Figure 6.43

around the glenoid component, but shoulder arthroscopy (Figures 6.42 and 6.43) with probing confirmed that the glenoid component was not loose from the scapula.

Shoulder sepsis

Another rare indication for shoulder arthroscopy is sepsis. The cannula can be used to wash out the shoulder joint copiously. The synovial appearance depends on the length of history but can be quite florid. Following washout of the joint, drains can be placed both from the anterior portal and up the arthroscope cannula prior to withdrawal, allowing a continuous irrigation system to be used postoperatively.

7 Arthroscopic surgery

Arthroscopic surgery of the shoulder is still very much in its infancy, but appears to be emerging at a virtually uncontrollable rate. When discussing such a new technique, two basic questions must be asked. The first is 'what *can* be achieved?' The second, and far more important, is 'what *should* be achieved?' For the wise surgeon will realize that the mere ability to perform an operation should not be an indication for its use. This chapter aims to answer both of these questions in turn, through a review of current techniques.

At present, arthroscopic surgery of the shoulder can be considered on five planes of increasing complexity, as shown in Table 7.1.

First generation surgery

First generation surgery is simple surgery that can be performed with the most basic equipment: an arthroscope, hook probe, basket forceps, and graspers.

Diagnostic arthroscopy

Diagnostic arthroscopy is by far the most important of the procedures in this group and has been covered in Chapters 4, 5 and 6.

Targeted biopsy

The indications for targeted biopsy are similar to those in the knee. The synovium of the shoulder may be affected by infection, either

Table 7.1 Five generations of arthroscopic surgery

First generation	Diagnostic arthroscopy Targeted biopsy Removal of loose bodies Excision of labral tears
Second generation	Synovectomy Shoulder debridement Coraco-acromial ligament division Arthroscopic subacromial decompression (ASD)
Third generation	Anterior reconstruction Staple Cannulated screw Rivet Suture
Fourth generation	Complex reconstruction SLAP tears Inferior capsular shift Combined intracapsular/ extracapsular repair
Fifth generation	Arthrodesis Rotator cuff repair

acute or chronic, specific and non-specific inflammation, crystal arthropathy, pigmented villonodular synovitis, and synovial chondromatosis. Specific to the synovium of the shoulder are superior synovial syndrome, a shoulder syndrome first described by Bayley (personal communication, 1989). In this condition there is a synovitis of the superior synovium alone, and biopsy has shown no increase in inflammatory cells. Frozen shoulder is a symptom complex rather than a syndrome[1] and the arthroscopic appearance can be extremely varied.[2] An example of this variance is shown in Figure 7.1. Both of these patients have the symptoms of frozen shoulder and yet the macroscopic pathology is totally different, with joint appearance normal in one and totally disorganized in the other.

Ogilvie Harris[3] reported his results on the arthroscopic management of frozen shoulder in 81 patients. All had spontaneous onset of shoulder pain and stiffness with no recognizable alternative pathology. However, at arthroscopy, 14 of the group were noted to have early osteoarthritis, 17 a partial thickness rotator cuff tear, and 11 were diabetic. All had a reduced joint capacity of around 20 ml. There was a mild synovitis in all cases, no obliteration of the infraglenoid recess and no adhesions, as had also been noted independently by Ha'eri[4] and Johnson[5]. The main pathology was contracture of the anterior capsular structures. In the first

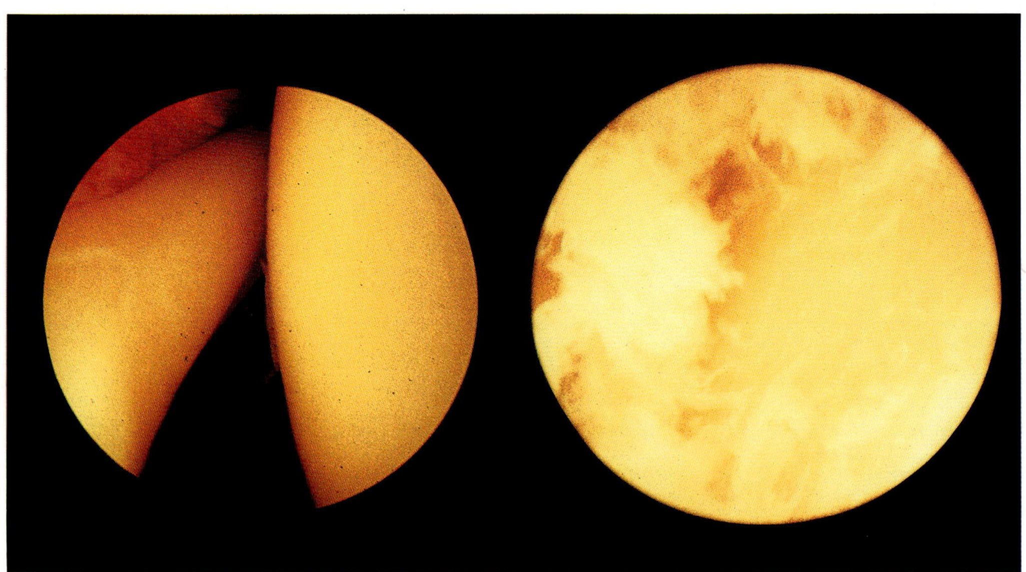

Figure 7.1

Both these patients have 'frozen shoulder'. However, macroscopically the shoulder arthroscopy shows a completely different pathology in each joint.

part of the series, arthroscopic joint distension was performed until the capsule ruptured. A manipulation was then performed and in some cases the joint was then rearthroscoped and the anterior capsule was found to be torn, revealing the subscapularis tendon. Of those patients with idiopathic frozen shoulder, 89 per cent had a successful result following this. However, success was measured in crude terms, and whether such a result would have occurred with manipulation alone is not known.

Biopsy can be performed either through the anterior portal, or through an accessory posterior portal. The anterior portal is best if the main area of synovial disease is in the superior part of the joint. If the disease is either in the infraglenoid recess or the posterior gutter, then an accessory posterior portal 2 cm below the posterior portal where the arthroscope lies, can be used. When using this portal, the position of the axillary nerve should be remembered.

Removal of loose bodies

Loose bodies are found in about 14 per cent of patients with recurrent dislocation;[5] may occur without dislocation in top class gymnasts,[6] or be associated with synovial chondromatosis.

As in the knee, removal of loose bodies may be challenging. They tend to gravitate to the lowermost recesses of the shoulder joint: the

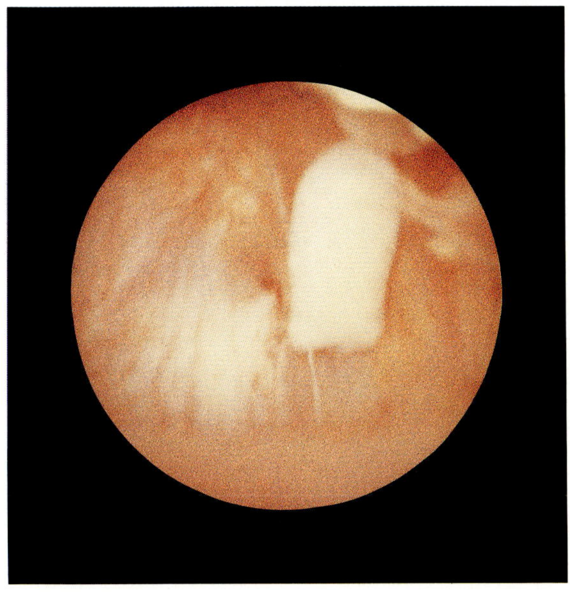

Figure 7.2

Loose bodies may be found in the infraglenoid recess.

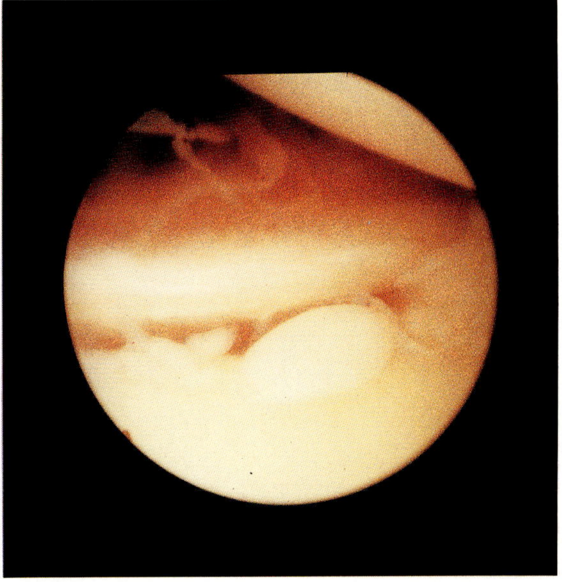

Figure 7.3

Another hiding place of loose bodies is the subscapular recess.

infraglenoid recess (Figure 7.2) and the subscapularis recess (Figure 7.3). Often these loose bodies are purely cartilaginous, having arisen from the impression fracture of the Hill–Sachs lesion. They will not therefore appear on the preoperative radiographs, but will appear later as an unexpected treat for the arthroscopist.

If the loose body is found in the infraglenoid recess, then it is best removed through an accessory posterior portal. A needle is first inserted through the portal and brought on to the loose body to assess the ability to remove the latter from that site (Figure 7.4). Having adjusted the needle placement to the best direction, the skin is incised at this point. A sharp trochar and cannula is then inserted into the joint to make a passage through the posterior capsule. The trochar and cannula are withdrawn and the grasping forceps inserted in the same direction until they lie next to the loose body (Figure 7.5). If, during any of these stages, bleeding starts to obscure the view, an irrigation needle should be inserted from the

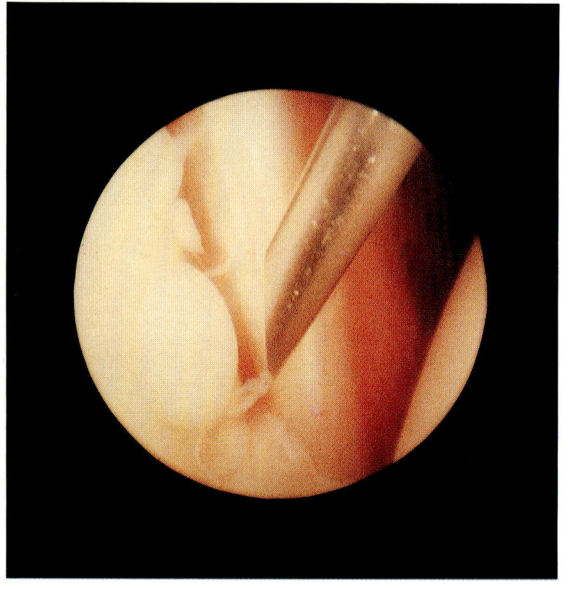

Figure 7.4

A needle is brought on to the loose body to assess the line for the grasping forceps.

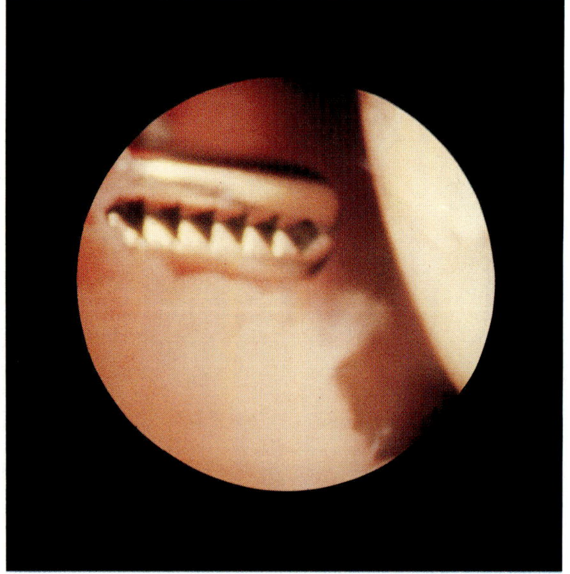

Figure 7.5

The grasping forceps is then brought on to the loose body which is removed.

anterior portal (Figure 7.6). The flow tends to disturb loose bodies less in the shoulder than the knee. The loose body is then grasped and withdrawn.

If the loose body is in the subscapularis recess, it may be difficult to see with a 30 degree arthroscope from the posterior portal. It is best then to change to a 70 degree arthroscope which can be advanced over the anterior edge of the glenoid to see down into the subscapularis recess. A needle is then inserted through the anterior portal to lie alongside the loose body, the track dilated with sharp trochar and cannula, the grasping forceps inserted down the track and the body grasped and removed.

Loose body removal is usually successful. Ogilvie Harris[3] described 11 cases, 3 associated with instability and 3 with osteoarthritis. In 10 cases, arthroscopic removal was successful, the one unsuccessful case being a large loose body in a recurrently dislocating shoulder, which was later successfully removed at open surgery.

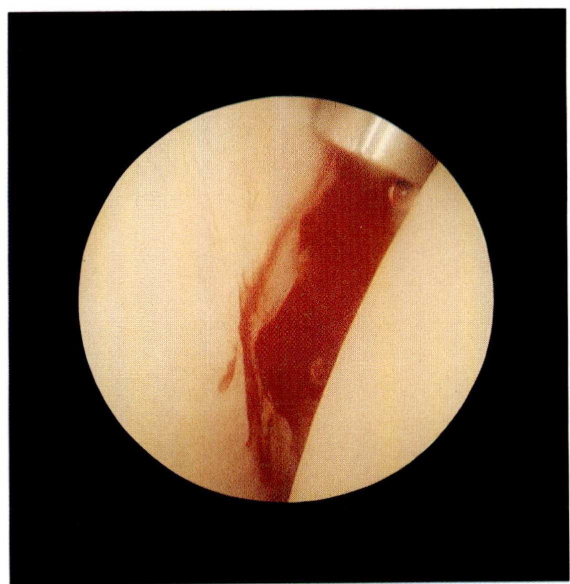

Figure 7.6
Bleeding can be cleared with a Verres needle.

Excision of labral tears

Tears of the glenoid labrum can be divided into two types, and the distinction is critical. The first is a tear of the superior anterior labrum, which is probably caused by avulsion of the superior labrum and biceps insertion during the deceleration phase of throwing, and is not associated with instability. The second is avulsion of the anteroinferior labrum caused by the subluxing or dislocating shoulder tearing away the portion of the labrum that forms the origin of the inferior glenohumeral ligament from the glenoid. The latter is the Bankart lesion and should never be excised (Figure 7.7).

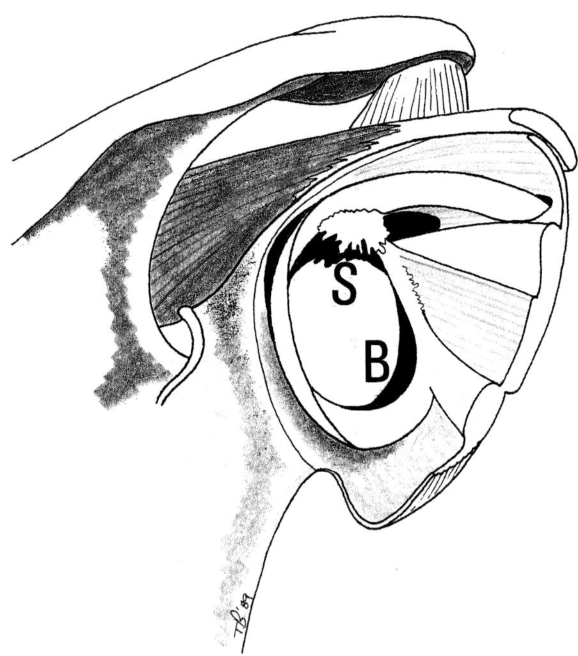

Figure 7.7

The superior labral tear must be differentiated from a Bankart lesion. Resection of a Bankart lesion will make the instability, and thus the patient's symptoms, worse.

Andrews et al[7] encountered 269 labral tears in 396 shoulders. About half were throwing athletes whose main complaints were pain (95 per cent) and popping (47 per cent) of the shoulder whilst throwing. Andrews has shown that, in these anterosuperior tears, the long head of biceps tears the glenoid labrum by traction upon it. This was confirmed when biceps was electrically stimulated during arthroscopy and was seen to pull the labrum and extend the tear.

The superior labrum may become quite degenerate and long tags may hang down between the humeral head and the glenoid. If a tear of this part of the labrum is seen and the surgeon is absolutely sure that the shoulder joint is stable and that the tear does not extend below the superior one-third of the anterior labrum, then the torn portion may be excised. The anterior portal is dilated up and the base of the tag can be cut through using the basket forceps, which can also be used to remove the tag from the joint. If the tear is extensively frayed, a full radius soft tissue resector may be used to excise the tear.

In Andrews' series,[7] 73 per cent of patients had an excellent result, 19 per cent a good result, and only 8 per cent a poor result. All athletes with excellent or good results returned to their throwing sport.

Second generation surgery

Whereas first generation surgery can be performed with minimal instrumentation, second generation surgery requires powered instruments. Arthroscopic subacromial decompression (ASD) also requires an electrosurgical diathermy apparatus to speed up the procedure and control bleeding, although many surgeons make do without.

Synovectomy

Synovectomy can be performed in rheumatoid arthritis, but is technically difficult due to bleeding and the results are as yet unknown. In Ogilvie Harris' series,[3] 12 of 15 patients undergoing synovectomy for rheumatoid arthritis had significant benefit at 1–2 years' follow-up.

Shoulder debridement

Osteoarthritis

Debridement can be performed in patients with mild osteoarthritis, a full radius resector being used to clean up the joint generally. In 43 patients in Ogilvie Harris' study,[3] 13 had mild arthritis and 69 per cent of these did well compared to only 37 per cent of the 30 with severe arthritis.

Cuff tears

Most surgeons would combine debridement of a cuff tear with subacromial decompression, and results of this are given in Chapter 8. The largest series of cuff debridement without decompression was again that of Ogilvie Harris,[3] who reported on 174 patients. In those patients with stage 1 impingement (tendonitis), 67 per cent were successful. However, in those patients with stage 2 (partial thickness tear) the results dropped to only 40 per cent successful and, in those with full thickness tears, the results fell even further to only 17 per cent successful results.

Coracoacromial ligament division

Most surgeons no longer perform coracoacromial ligament division alone, but instead arthroscopic subacromial decompression. Ogilvie Harris[3] published his group's results from division alone in 51 patients, 25 of whom had mechanical division and 26 electrocautery division. As only 11 of the 51 patients had a satisfactory outcome, the group concluded that this procedure should be abandoned.

Arthroscopic subacromial decompression (ASD)

This is covered in more detail in Chapter 8, pages 133–142.

Third and fourth generation surgery

These techniques are discussed in Chapter 9.

Fifth generation surgery

Arthrodesis

Arthrodesis is technically feasible. Here, both the glenoid and humerus are burred down to subchondral bone, and percutaneous screws are placed, backed up with an external fixator. However, the only attempt to this date has been unsuccessful. Such technical feats show a lack of maturity and wisdom on the part of the surgeon.

Rotator cuff repair

Successful rotator cuff repair has been performed, but the patient selection is critical. The technique can only be performed on *small* rotator cuff tears. The tear is assessed and the edges are debrided. The area where the torn-off cuff should insert is then burred down until there is bleeding from the bone surface. The debrided cuff is then impaled with an arthroscopic staple, which is advanced onto the prepared bed and hammered into the humeral head. At 6 weeks the staple is retrieved arthroscopically and the cuff assessed to see if healing has occurred. If there is impingement at this stage, subacromial decompression can be carried out.

It must be stressed that this is an unproven technique at this stage with no follow up reports in the literature. The wise surgeon will await the results from those centres pioneering these techniques.

8 Arthroscopic subacromial decompression

Impingement

Our understanding of the impingement syndrome has greatly improved over the past few years and there is no doubt that this will continue for the next decade. It is becoming apparent that impingement is just the final common pathway for a number of different pathologies. Perhaps the best way to look at impingement is anatomically and functionally.

The subacromial space is not a true space but a *potential* space. Thus it has a roof and a floor, but no real walls. This potential space is lined by the subacromial bursa. The subacromial space is roofed by the acromion, the acromioclavicular joint, the extreme distal portion of the clavicle, the coracoacromial ligament and, anteriorly, the coracoid process itself. The floor of the space is the rotator cuff, the coracohumeral ligament and the long head of biceps. Once distended, the potential space becomes a space: the anterior wall consists of the coracoid process, the lateral and posterior walls are formed by the deltoid and the medial wall is made of bands from the coracoacromial ligament to the acromioclavicular joint and the musculotendinous junction of supraspinatus (Figure 8.1).

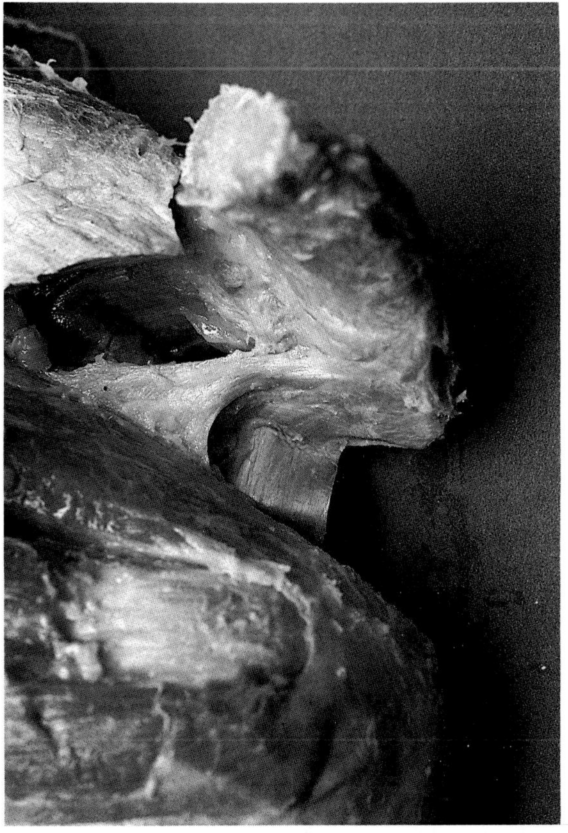

Figure 8.1
Anatomy of the subacromial space.

The subacromial space can therefore be compromised either by the roof coming down, or the floor coming up. The roof can only come down by some part of it being thicker anatomically, but the floor can come up both anatomically (by a thickening of the floor), or functionally (by upward subluxation of the glenohumeral joint, which can be physiological or pathological).

A 'lower' roof

The acromion

The shape of the anterior acromion varies from person to person, and may be flat or hooked. The Bigliani classification recognizes three types of shape, varying from flat (type 1) to fully hooked (type 3). The best way to appreciate the acromial shape is to take a subacromial arch radiograph. The relevance of the Bigliani type 3 acromion is that the hook will have to be surgically excised.

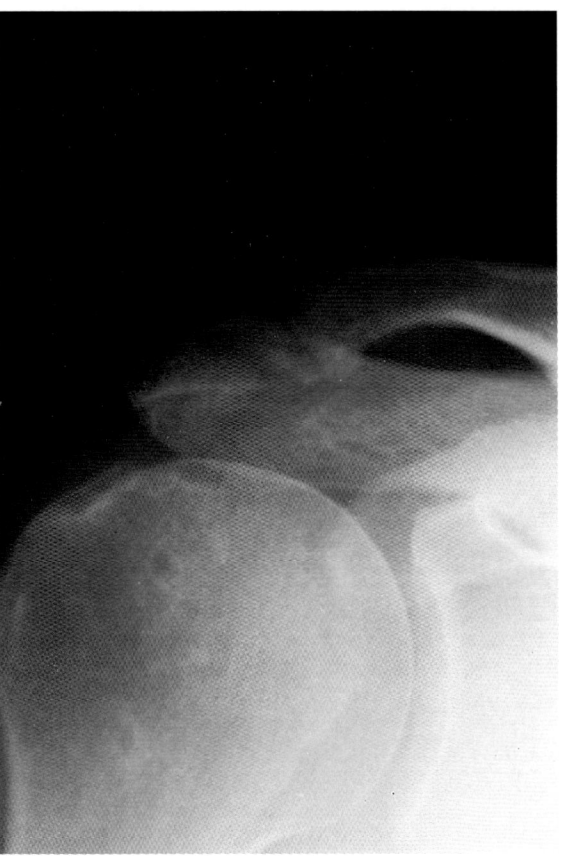

Figure 8.2
Inferior osteophytes projecting down from the acromioclavicular joint.

The acromioclavicular joint

Figures vary but, on average, 30 per cent of patients with impingement will have degenerate changes visible in the acromioclavicular joint on an anteroposterior radiograph of the shoulder. A proportion of these will have inferior osteophytes (Figure 8.2) projecting down into the subacromial space. The capsule of the acromioclavicular joint may also be thickened. Obviously, to remove the osteophytes, the capsule has to be resected first.

The coracoacromial ligament

We have already shown that the coracoacromial ligament inserts *underneath* the acromion and not onto the front of the acromion, so any thickening of this ligament at its insertion point will project into the subacromial space.

The coracoid process

Gerber et al[1] have described a variety of anterior impingement caused by the proximity of the coracoid to the front of the shoulder, which is relieved by the operation of coracoplasty.

A 'higher' floor (anatomical)

Rotator cuff

The rotator cuff can be thickened either due to a partial thickness tear, with the torn ends hanging into the joint, or by a deposit within the tendon such as calcific tendinitis. The retracted end of a full thickness tear may roll up, thereby decreasing the space.

Thickening of the bursa

The bursa may be thickened secondary to any abnormality of the subacromial space and will further decrease the space available.

A 'higher' floor (functional)

Physiological

Matthews and Fadale[2] have shown how the subacromial space is diminished with abduction of the arm. Sigholm et al,[3] using a microcapillary infusion technique, have measured the pressure in the subacromial space. At rest, the pressure was 8 mmHg, rising to 32 mmHg with the arm abducted to 45 degrees and to 56 mmHg with the arm abducted to 45 degrees while holding a 1 kg weight. This 'physiological impingement' has relevance both to work-related and sport-related impingement.

Pathological

Upward subluxation of the glenohumeral joint may be caused by instability, or by an abnormality of muscular or nervous control of the rotator cuff. In particular, rotator cuff tears can lead to upward subluxation (Figure 8.3). Weakness of the rotator cuff, secondary to suprascapular nerve entrapment, may cause upward subluxation.

Obviously an understanding of the aetiology of impingement is vital to the correct management. For instance, if a particular patient has impingement secondary to instability, then the capsule should be repaired. Subacromial decompression will only make this patient worse. A patient with anterior impingement between the cuff and the coracoid needs a coracoplasty and will not get better with a subacromial decompression. A patient with work-related physiological impingement may need only to change his posture, for example, to working with the elbow at the side instead of abducted. Patient selection is the key to success with subacromial decompression.[4]

Natural history of impingement

Neer[5] classified the impingement syndrome into three stages according to changes in the rotator cuff, caused by repeated abrasion against the roof of the subacromial space. Stage 1 causes oedema and haemorrhage in the cuff, occurs in the younger patient, is often work- or sport-related and tends to settle with conservative measures. Stage 2 causes fibrosis and 'tendinitis' or partial thickness tears, occurs in an older age group and is more resistant to therapy. Stage 3 implies full thickness rotator cuff tears, rupture of the biceps tendon and bone changes.

Chard et al[6] reviewed 137 patients with impingement treated conservatively. At a mean of over 18 months, 35 still had active tendinitis, a further 40 still had residual pain and 8 had developed pain due to other causes. Only 54 resolved and these were distinguished by early presentation and a history of overuse unrelated to occupation. In 29 patients, function was still impaired and 2 lost their jobs. Chard and colleagues concluded that rotator cuff tendinitis

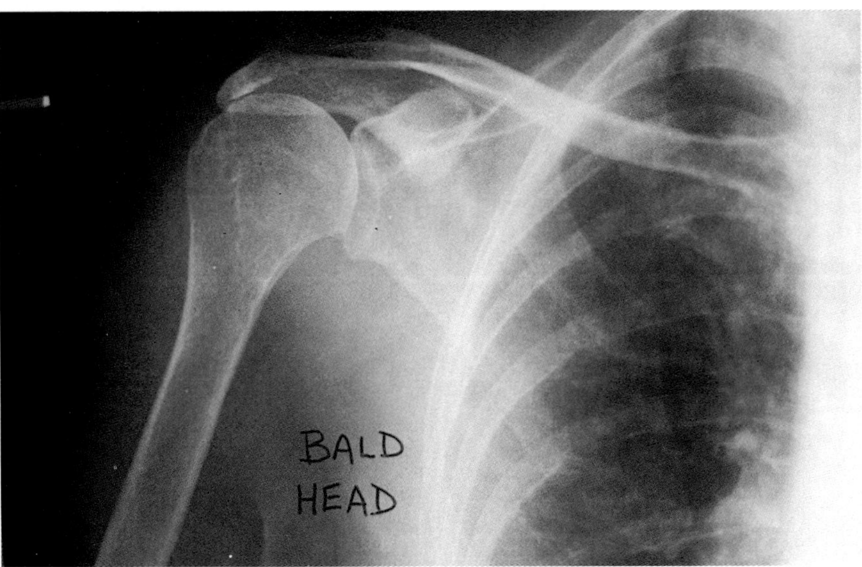

Figure 8.3
Upward subluxation of the humeral head following rotator cuff tear.

is not an early self-limiting condition, that a sizeable proportion did not resolve with conservative management and that improvements in management were needed.

Indications for surgery

For open or closed surgery, the diagnosis of impingement must be watertight, subluxation must have been excluded, the patient must be over 35 years, must have failed to respond to conservative management, and must have had the symptoms in excess of 6 months, with no improvement.

Diagnosis

A scheme for diagnosis is given in the algorithm shown in Figure 8.4. The patient will typically be a man of over 40 years who complains of true shoulder pain, which is exacerbated in the mid-range of elevation, a mid-range painful arc. The onset is usually insidious. If there is a history of trauma, then cuff tear and dislocation or subluxation should be excluded. If the painful arc is work- or sport-related then it may be physiological and a change in posture may be of benefit during working or sporting activities. Unfortunately, most patients will have worked this out for themselves before attending a surgeon and have not achieved success.

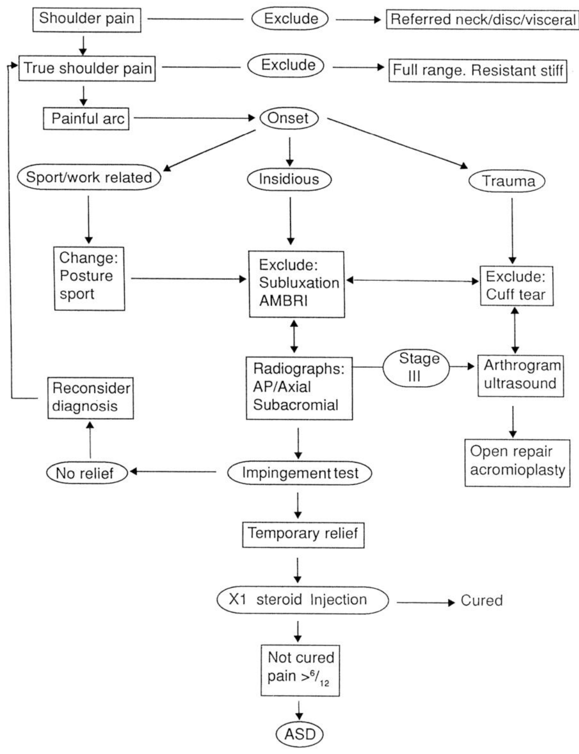

Figure 8.4

Diagnostic algorithm for impingement.

During the examination, particular attention should be paid to the tests for dislocation, the apprehension tests, sulcus sign and any joint laxity. If there is pain on cross-body adduction, attention should be paid to the acromioclavicular joint and the coracoid. If subcoracoid impingement is suspected, a CT scan should be performed. If there is excessive muscle wasting or weakness, the surgeon should suspect a cuff tear or neurological cause.

Three plain radiographs should be taken, an anteroposterior view of the shoulder, an axial and a subacromial arch view. If there are bone changes on the anteroposterior view (cysts or sclerosis of the greater tuberosity, sclerosis of the undersurface of the acromion, or a decrease in the acromiohumeral interval below 7 mm) then the patient has stage 3 impingement or cuff tear and is a poor candidate for arthroscopic treatment. Degenerative change in the acromioclavicular joint with inferior spikes means that the outer 1 cm of the clavicle may need to be excised, and this is best done with open surgery. If the arch view shows a Bigliani type 3 acromion, then a bony procedure must be performed.

The 'impingement test' should now be performed, 2 ml 1 per cent lignocaine (US: lidocaine) being injected just under the anterior acromion. The patient is re-examined at 5 minutes and, for a diagnosis of impingement to hold good, the patient's painful arc should have improved dramatically.

If the patient has had no previous conservative treatment and the time course is under 6 months' duration, then a single steroid injection of 40 mg depomedrone, or equivalent dosage of triamcinalone, may be injected under the anterior acromion, the patient being re-examined in 6 weeks. If the patient fails to respond to conservative measures, then surgery can be considered.

Open or closed surgery?

Before electing for closed surgery, both surgeon and patient must be convinced of its superiority over open surgery. Presently this is debatable.

The method of open surgery has been described by Neer:[5] 2 cm of anterior deltoid are released from the anterior acromion and the coracoacromial ligament and anteroinferior acromion are excised. Any osteophytes under the acromioclavicular joint are excised and the rotator cuff is checked for evidence of tears. The deltoid is then carefully reattached and the skin closed. Hawkins[4] reviewed 108 patients who underwent open acromioplasty, and who had no cuff tear. All patients had shoulder pain for over 1 year before operation, despite conservative treatment. Open acromioplasty was successful in 87 per cent of patients. The operation was less successful in women, those with limited preoperative movement, those who were involved in work compensation, and those whose pain had started after direct trauma. In most surgeons' hands, closed acromioplasty is not as successful as this, although the recent results of Ellman and Kay[7] at 85 per cent satisfactory for stage 2 impingement and of Alcheck et al[8] at 82 per cent excellent and good are comparable.

There is no doubt that arthroscopic subacromial decompression (ASD) is both more difficult and generally takes longer than open procedure. Although ASD has these drawbacks, and tends not to be as successful as open acromioplasty, it does have advantages. These are that it is a day-case procedure, for some reason it is less painful, and the patient has faster rehabilitation. There is no doubt that arthroscopic surgery has a good image amongst the population at large and, to an extent, the patient now demands minimally invasive surgery if possible.

ASD Ellman method

Equipment

Many surgeons perform ASD with powered shaver systems alone. However, the soft tissue covering under the acromion (the insertion of the coracoacromial ligament) is very resistant to a powered resector, and virtually immune to a burr, as it is firm and rubbery. This means that electrosurgical apparatus is really necessary and cuts surgical time considerably.

Method

The patient is placed in the lateral position, prepared, draped and a shoulder arthroscopy is performed. The arthroscope is then placed in the subacromial bursa (see Chapter 5). Ellman[9] suggests that the posterior portal is used for an inflow and that the arthroscope is inserted 1 cm below and 1 cm anterior to the posterior angle of the acromion (Figure 8.5).

Two 18-gauge spinal needles are now inserted to outline the anterior border of the acromion (Figure 8.6). The medial needle is placed just in front of the acromioclavicular joint and the lateral needle in front of the anterolateral angle of the acromion.

The soft tissue must now be removed from the undersurface of the acromion, and this means that the coracoacromial ligament must be divided. Ogilvie Harris (personal communication, 1988) has examined the blood supply of the coracoacromial ligament in cadavers. He has shown that the largest vessels are at the coracoid end. At the midway point there are usually three vessels in the ligament, but only 1 in 20 had a blood vessel within 1 cm of the insertion of the ligament. The entry point for the instruments is 3–4 cm from the acromion, in direct line with the two pins (Figure 8.7). The coracoacromial ligament is divided from the medial marker pin to the lateral marker pin, using the electrosurgical apparatus (Figure 8.3). For the electrosurgical apparatus to function, the saline must be flushed out of the bursa and sterile distilled water for irrigation must be instilled.

Once the coracoacromial ligament has been divided, the area of resection should be circumscribed, using the electrosurgical apparatus (Figure 8.9). The tissue within this circle is

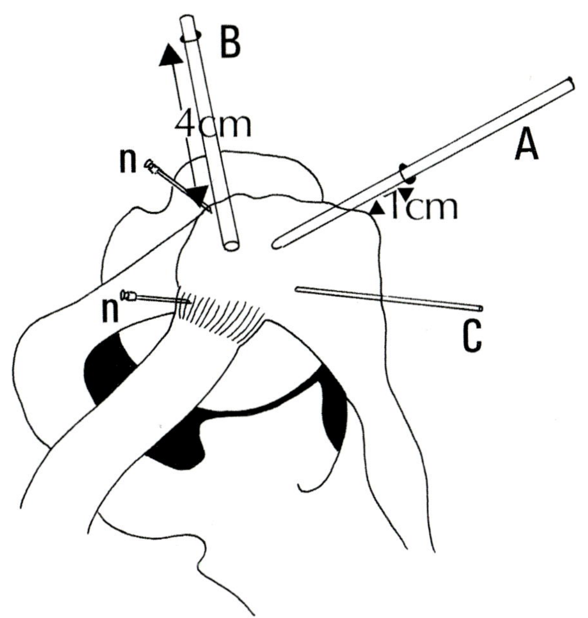

Figure 8.5

Portals for arthroscopic subacromial decompression.

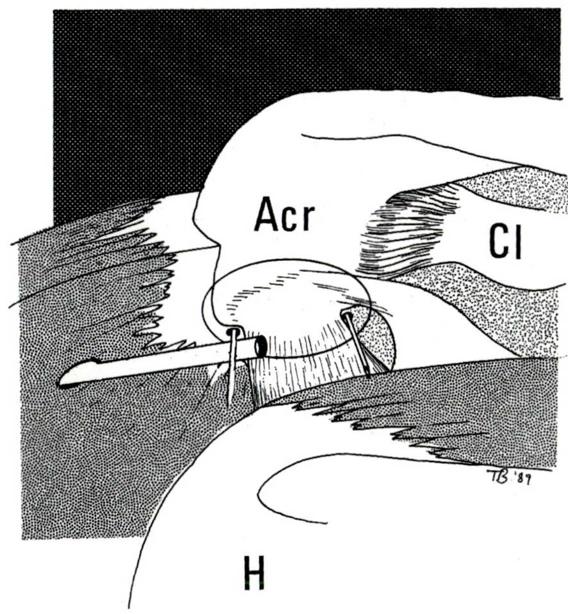

Figure 8.7

The entry point for the instruments is 3–4 cm from the acromion in direct line with the two pins.

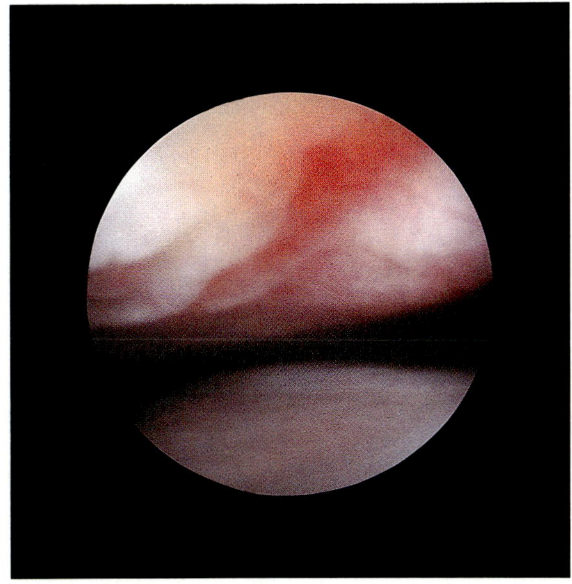

Figure 8.6

Needles are inserted to mark the edges of the coracoacromial ligament.

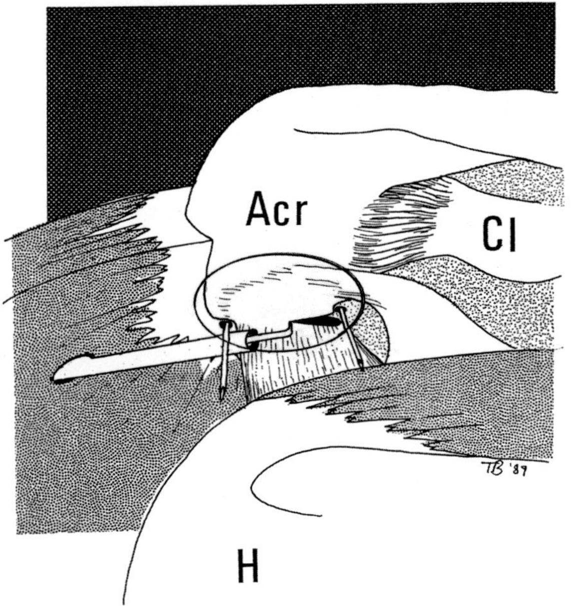

Figure 8.8

The coracoacromial ligament is divided with the electrosurgical apparatus.

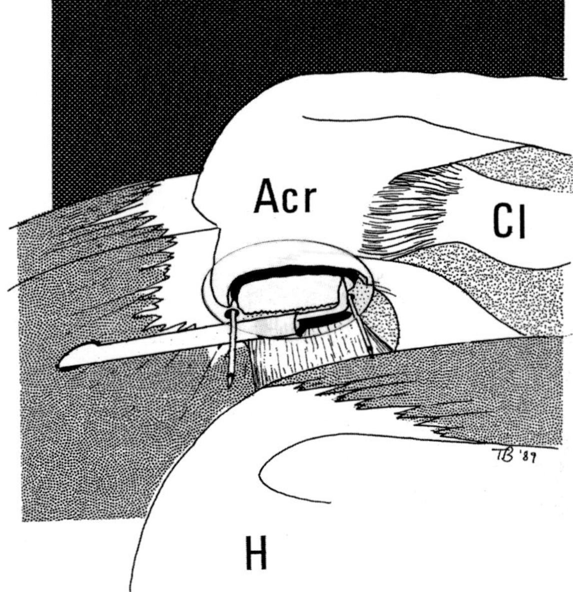

Figure 8.9

The area for resection is circumscribed by the electrosurgical apparatus.

then morsellized with the cutting diathermy so that it hangs down in strips.

The electrosurgical apparatus is now exchanged for the powered full radius resector and all the morsellized tissue resected so that the undersurface of the bone can be seen (Figure 8.10). The full radius resector is now exchanged for an acromionizer burr and the acromioplasty started. Ellman recommends that the burring starts from the anteromedial corner of the acromion, with a deepening hole 3 mm deep which is then extended as a trough from front to back for a distance of 2.5 cm. Further troughs are now made across the width of the acromion (Figure 8.11). Finally the whole area is polished by circular passes of the burr and the process repeated until the required depth is achieved.

Osteophyte under the acromioclavicular joint should be resected and this requires removal of the inferior capsule before the bone can be burred away.

As in any surgical procedure, the key is visualization, and this is the problem with ASD. Firstly, the surgeon is working in a restricted space and, secondly, the tissues tend to bleed.

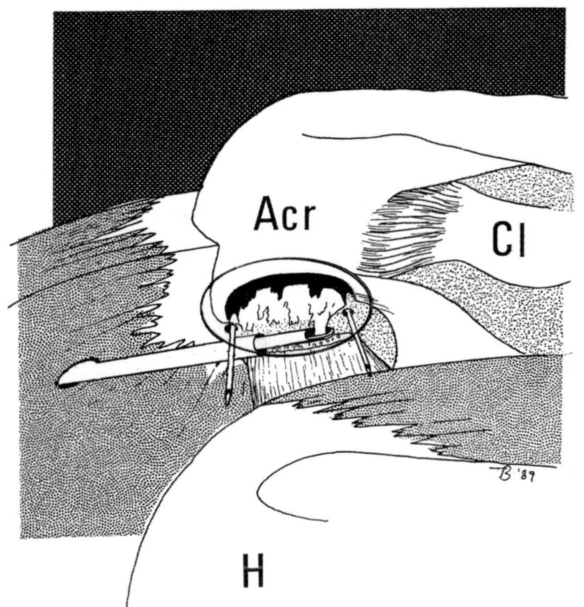

Figure 8.10

The full radius resector is used to remove the soft tissue under the acromion.

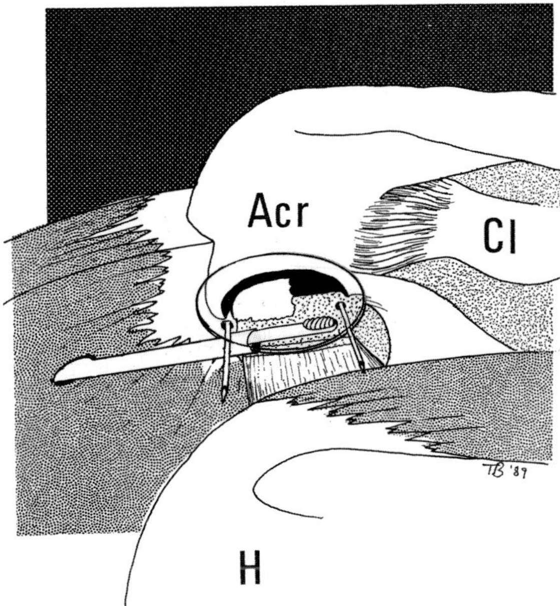

Figure 8.11

The acromionizer burr is then used to resect the undersurface of the acromion.

Thirdly, the soft tissue does not peel away cleanly and the surgeon finds himself performing an arthroscopic procedure amongst dense seaweed in extremely murky water. Access can be improved by traction of the limb in a caudad manner with a shoulder holder, but the arm must be kept at the side and not abducted as this restricts vision. High pressure irrigation must be used. This does not necessarily mean an infusion pump, although many surgeons find this helps, but there must be adequate flow, under adequate pressure, which means a high head of pressure, a high drip stand and wide-bore inflow tubing. As already stated, an electrosurgical apparatus cuts down bleeding and operation time considerably.

Postoperative management

The shoulder swells to an alarming extent following this procedure but this tends to reduce within hours. A sling should not be worn. The patient should perform pendulum exercises every morning and every evening for 1 minute. Strenuous overhead activities, such as tennis and throwing, should be avoided for at least 4–6 weeks. At 6 weeks, strengthening exercises are begun.

Results

Ellman described his 2–5 year results at the American Academy of Orthopaedic Surgeons' meeting in 1989.[7] He started ASD in 1985 and performed 10 cases in that year. By 1987 he had performed 50 cases and by 1989 217 cases. He reported on the 87 cases with a follow-up of 2–5 years. Of these, 79 per cent had stage 2 impingement and 21 per cent had stage 3 – that is, a full thickness cuff tear. The average follow-up was 34 months and the average age 49 years. The patients had received on average four steroid injections prior to surgery and nearly all had experienced night pain. The patients were assessed using UCLA scores and 85 per cent were satisfactory, 76 per cent returning to sport. Of the patients with stage 2 impingement, 89 per cent were satisfactory, but those with cuff tears had worse results, only 65 per cent being satisfactory. The group with cuff tears had an average age of 74 years and Ellman believes that open treatment is preferable to ASD if a cuff tear is present.

Gartsman also presented his results at this meeting.[10] He showed that results in stage 2 impingement were good, 88 per cent being satisfied, but this dropped to 82.5 per cent satisfaction in the face of a partial thickness tear, and fell even further to only 45 per cent satisfaction in the presence of a full thickness tear.

Warren et al[11] presented results in 40 patients undergoing ASD and debridement of the acromioclavicular joint under scalene block, performed between 1984 and 1986. Of these, 20 had stage 2 impingement and 10 stage 3. The average age was 43 years. All had a glenohumeral arthroscopy and 31 abnormalities were found, 11 had labral pathology, 10 had full thickness tears, three had partial thickness tears and seven had tendinitis of the long head of the biceps. Overall, 80 per cent were excellent or good as rated by the Hospital for Special Surgery (HSS) scoring system, 14 per cent were fair and 16 per cent poor. The average time to recovery was 3.8 months, most were in work at 10 days and 77 per cent returned to their premorbidity sporting level. Five of the six who failed to return to sport had anteroinferior labral tears (Bankart lesions). Warren stresses that impingement secondary to instability should not be treated by ASD and that patients with moderate size tears should have these repaired at open surgery.

9 Arthroscopic management of traumatic shoulder dislocation

Background

Shoulder dislocation can be classified into one of two types:

- TUBS: Traumatic, Unidirectional, Bankart, Surgery
- AMBRI: Atraumatic, Multidirectional, Bilateral, Rehabilitation, Shift[1]

The great majority of TUBS are anterior dislocations (98 per cent in Rowe's[2] series of 500), in whom a Bankart lesion is present in 85 per cent. The treatment of recurrence in this group is surgery.

AMBRI is a smaller group, usually initiated without trauma, often multidirectional (anterior, inferior and posterior), occurring in patients with generalized joint laxity, the opposite shoulder usually being loose and demonstrating a sulcus sign. These patients *should not be operated upon*. Treatment initially consists of a programme of supervised shoulder strengthening exercises. If the shoulder does not respond to such a programme, the patient should be referred on to a shoulder specialist to consider a capsular shift operation. There is no place for arthroscopic repair in these patients.

Two large studies have been performed on the incidence of recurrent dislocation following traumatic anterior dislocation (Figure 9.1). We have already seen (Chapter 6, pages 99–124)

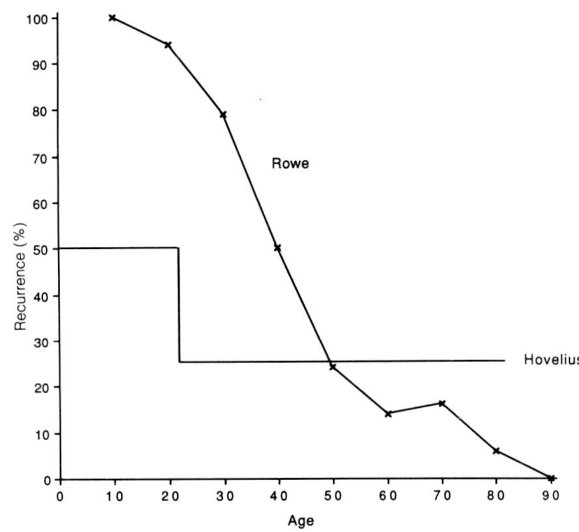

Figure 9.1

Incidence of recurrence following dislocation according to age at first dislocation. Data from Rowe and Hovelius.[2,3]

that there is a spectrum of both Bankart lesions (Figure 9.2) and Hill–Sachs lesions (Figure 9.3), and it is likely that the severity of damage to the anterior capsular structures is related to the number of recurrent dislocations.

A concept of anterior traumatic dislocation is where the aim of surgery is to identify precisely the pathology responsible for dislocation and to perform a selective repair: 'Not all shoulder instabilities are created equal, nor are they treated the same' (Johnson[4]).

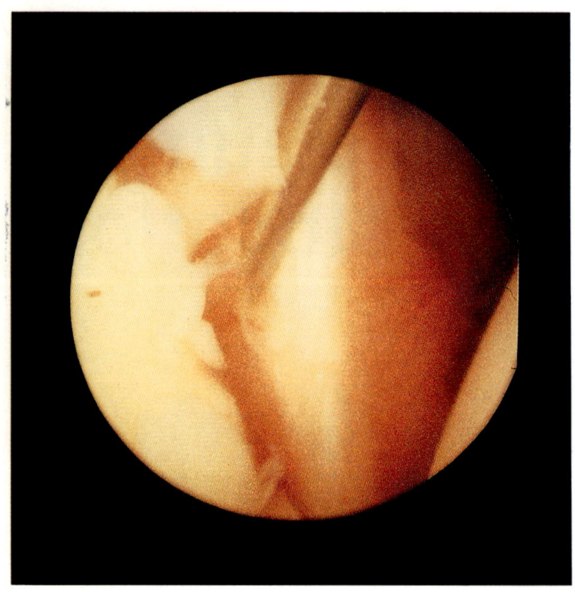

Figure 9.2
Bankart lesion of the glenoid labrum IGHL complex.

Recurrent anterior dislocation: pathological basis

The classic paper on stabilizing mechanisms preventing anterior dislocation of the glenohumeral joint by Turkel et al[5] should be read by all orthopaedic surgeons with an interest in shoulder dislocation. Turkel performed studies on 46 cadaveric shoulders with selective sectioning of the anterior structures to identify the relative contribution of each to shoulder instability, in various positions of the shoulder. The shoulder joints were opened posteriorly and wire sutures were inserted to mark the superior border of the middle glenohumeral ligament (MGHL), the superior and inferior margins of the thickening of the anterior inferior glenohumeral ligament (AIGHL) and the superior and inferior margins of the subscapularis muscle (marked from in front). Radiographs were then taken with the shoulder at 0, 45 and 90 degrees of abduction in external rotation (Figure 9.4). They concluded that at 0 degrees of abduction, anterior dislocation is prevented largely by subscapularis but, as the shoulder reaches 90 degrees abduction in external rotation (the position of apprehension), then the subscapularis rolls over the top of the humeral head and its inferior margin rides up exposing the lower half of the anterior surface of the head. The AIGHL was tight in this position and was the only structure covering the vulnerable antero-inferior portion of the humeral head.

In the selective cutting experiments, section of subscapularis alone did not allow subluxation or dislocation. When all the structures except the AIGHL had been sectioned, dislocation did not occur. However, as soon as the superior band of the AIGHL was sectioned, subluxation or dislocation did occur, and this increased as the axillary fold of the AIGHL was sectioned. A further selective cutting experiment division of the AIGHL alone, with all other structures intact, led to dislocation. These studies show the vital role of the AIGHL complex.

Anatomically we have seen that the anterior labrum is an extension of the AIGHL complex, and the Bankart lesion is an avulsion of the

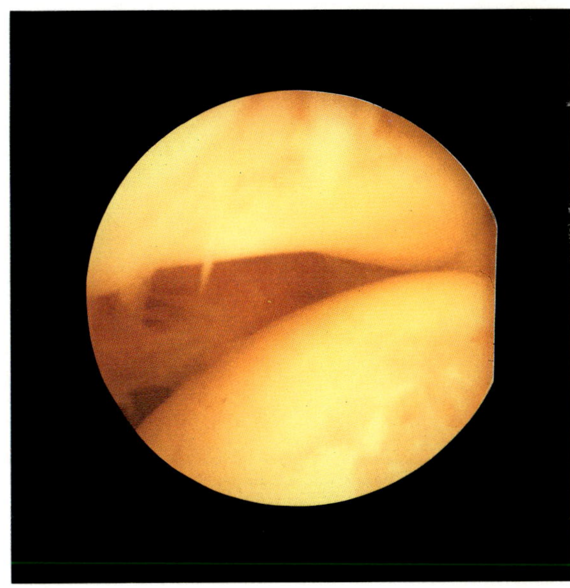

Figure 9.3

Hill–Sachs osteochondral lesion in the back of the humeral head.

AIGHL complex from its origin on the scapula. O'Brien and colleagues[6] have drawn attention to the role of the posterior band of the IGHL, and have shown how the IGHL can be likened to a hammock upon which the humeral head rests (see Figure 5.26). The Bankart lesion can be likened to section of one of the ropes supporting the hammock, and thus the head falls forward (Figure 9.5). Oveison and Nielson[7] have shown that a large lesion of the posterior capsule is needed for anterior dislocation and puts forward the concept of the capsule as a ring, the anterior part of which can only break if the posterior section comes forward as well.

In the 10–15 per cent of patients who are not shown to have a Bankart lesion, two factors must be considered. The first is that the diagnosis is incorrect, these patients may in fact be AMBRI with a lax AIGHL, in which case they must not undergo arthroscopic repair (Figure 9.6). The second is that the diagnosis of recurrent TUBS is correct but there has been

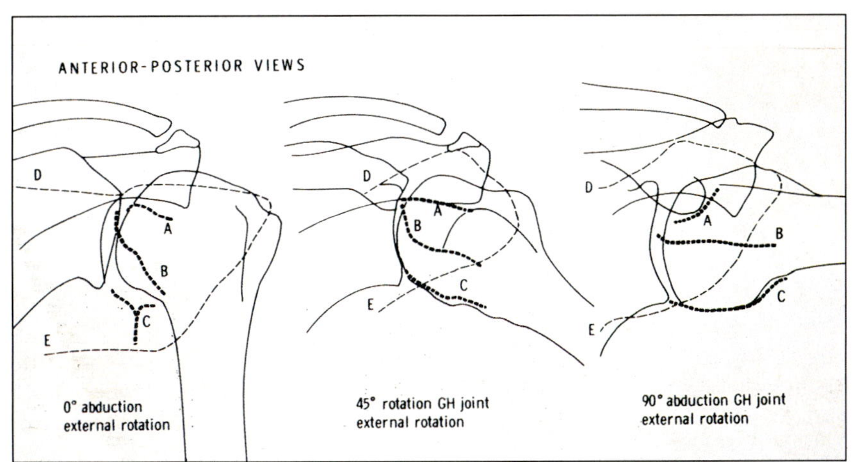

Figure 9.4

Position of the subscapularis (lines D and E), middle glenohumeral ligament (top margin is marked A) and inferior glenohumeral ligament (lines B and C), with the arm at the side, at 45 degrees of abduction and at 90 degrees of abduction and external rotation (the position of apprehension). (From Turkel et al.[5])

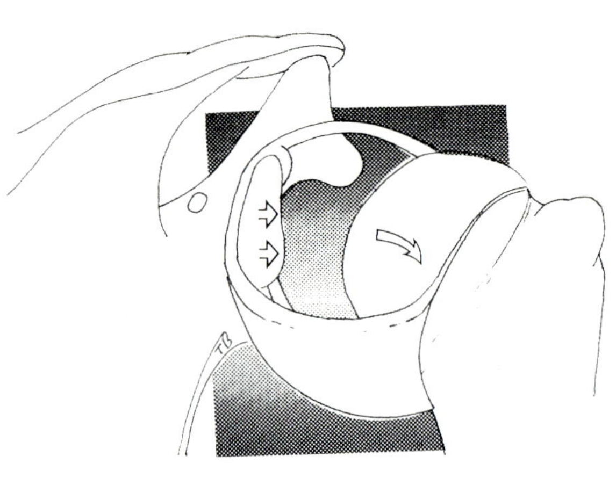

Figure 9.5

O'Brien et al[6] have described the inferior glenohumeral ligament/labral complex as a hammock, upon which the head lies. When the front supporting rope of the hammock is cut then the humeral head falls 'out of bed'.

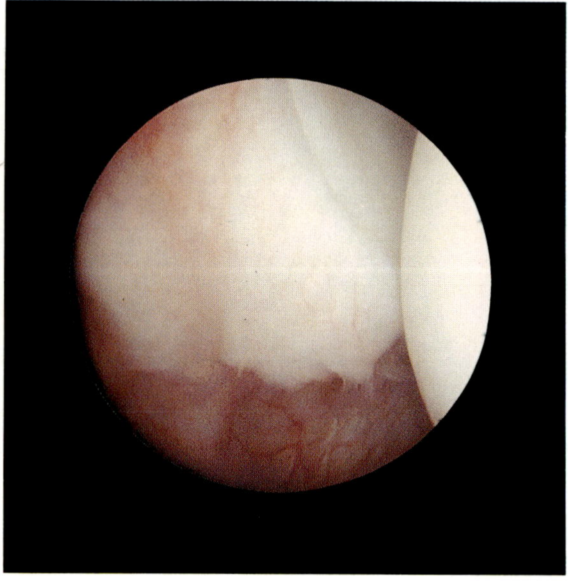

Figure 9.6

Multidirectional instability. Note the inferior shift of the humeral head so that its equator has almost slipped over the inferior glenoid into the infraglenoid recess.

plastic deformation, or stretching of the AIGHL rather than avulsion from its origin and these patients will need an inferior capsular shift.

Concerning the relevance of the Hill–Sachs lesion to recurrent TUBS, it should be recalled that the Hill–Sachs lesion is a *result* of the dislocation and not a cause of it. It is an impaction fracture of the dislocated head against the anterior glenoid. The only relevance of the Hill–Sachs lesion to the arthroscopic surgeon is that, if the defect is massive, then consideration should be given to a Connolly procedure (placing the insertion of infraspinatus within the defect), or a rotational osteotomy, rather than arthroscopic repair.

Fracture of the glenoid rim is a further contraindication to arthroscopic repair. The defect should be selectively repaired, which may mean a bony operation to restore the anterior glenoid. However, it should be said at this point that such a massive defect is rarely encountered. Minor crevassing of the anterior glenoid rim (Figure 9.7) is not a contraindication to arthroscopic repair.

Unfortunately, by the time patients are referred for surgery, they have often had multiple episodes of recurrent dislocation, and what may have started as a simple avulsion of the

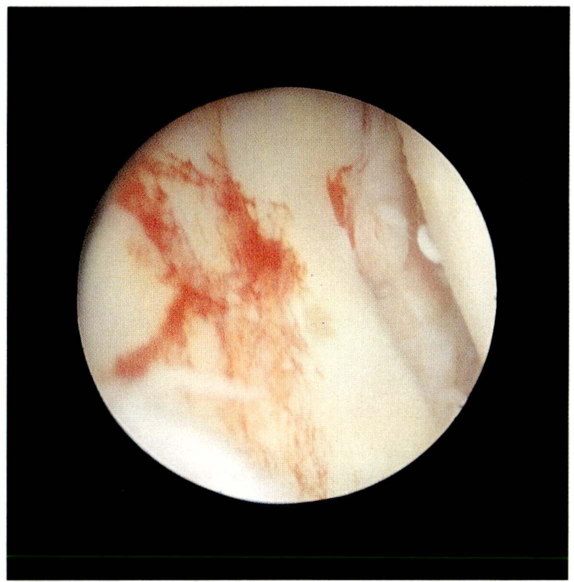

Figure 9.7
Crevassing of the anterior glenoid rim.

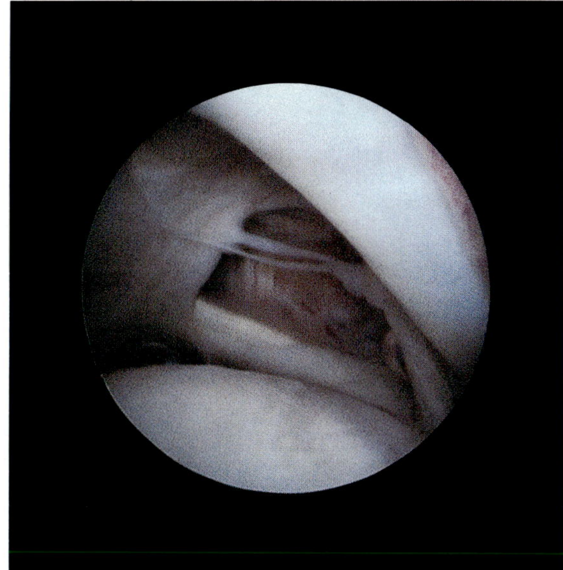

Figure 9.8
The labrum has been traumatized so much that it has disappeared from a long segment of the anterior glenoid.

AIGHL complex (Bankart lesion) undergoes repeated trauma, the Bankart lesion extends, the labrum fibrillates and tears within its substance and eventually disintegrates so that there is no trace left of it or the middle or inferior glenohumeral ligaments (Figure 9.8). Arthroscopic repair of the Bankart lesion is now impossible, and although Caspari's group have performed arthroscopic augmentations, the less experienced arthroscopic surgeon should abort the arthroscopy and move on to selective open repair. To abort an arthroscopic procedure is a sign of wisdom on the part of the surgeon, *not* an admission of failure.

Arthroscopic staple repair

On 14 September 1982, Johnson performed the first arthroscopic repair for anterior dislocation of the shoulder at Ingham Medical Center, Lansing, Michigan (Johnson LL, Detrisac DA, personal communication, 1983). The patient had sustained a traumatic anterior dislocation 6 months previously, with 100 subsequent dislocations, four in the week prior to surgery. After arthroscopic preparation of the anterior glenoid rim, the Bankart lesion was repaired using a specially devised staple, which was introduced through the anterior arthroscopic portal. By 1987, 195 repairs had been performed at Ingham Medical.

Although Perthes first used staples to repair the detached anterior capsule in 1906, the technique was popularized by Du Toit and Roux from Johannesburg.[8] They reported on an open staple repair which they had been performing since 1932. They credited the procedure to Fouche and Allen whose surgical staples were fashioned from bicycle spokes. The anatomical basis is to reattach the avulsed AIGHL labrum complex to the glenoid neck with the staple. The method was modified by Boyd and Hunt[9] who introduced a barbed staple. The simple nature of this open operation led to great popularity, but loosening of the staples and degenerative lesions of the glenoid rim have led to its discontinuation as an operation.

The simplicity of this open procedure led to its reintroduction by Johnson as an arthroscopic technique in 1982.[4] A special 4 mm staple was devised for arthroscopic delivery. The method according to Johnson is described below.

Method

Examination under anaesthesia

Both shoulders should be examined using the tests for instability (see Chapter 3). Johnson has found that external rotation is limited in the dislocating shoulder preoperatively by 12 degrees (with the elbow at the side) compared to the unaffected shoulder.

The patient is positioned in the lateral position for shoulder arthroscopy, and a single shoulder holder is used to suspend the arm. If the arm rolls into external rotation and starts to sublux in the suspension apparatus, then the procedure may become more than usually difficult. No more than 15 lb of traction should be used, as further traction can cause damage to the brachial plexus.

Diagnostic arthroscopy

The shoulder must *always* be arthroscoped prior to any surgical procedure for instability. Firstly, the joint can be examined far more thoroughly than at arthrotomy, allowing precise identification of the pathology, which in turn allows the surgeon to plan the selective repair required. For instance, a simple Bankart lesion needs a Bankart repair, either arthroscopic or open. A stretched AIGHL requires an open inferior capsular shift, and a patient with no labrum or glenohumeral ligaments needs an extra-articular augmentation, such as a Putti-Platt or Magnusson-Stack procedure.

Secondly, a large proportion of patients will have second pathology (Table 9.1) which can be assessed or corrected. Finally, the surgeon is given a legitimate reason for shoulder arthroscopy. The dislocating shoulder is ideal for training in shoulder arthroscopy as the joint is usually of large capacity, entry is easy, and there is a large amount of abnormal pathology on view.

Table 9.1 Associated lesions found during staple anterior repair (Johnson[4]).

n = 195	
13%	Cuff tear
90%	Hill–Sachs
4%	Anterior glenoid fracture
14%	Loose body
10%	Posterior labral tear

Exposure

The key to any surgical procedure is good exposure and this is as true of arthroscopy as of any open technique. Correct scope positioning, atraumatic single insertion, and joint distension are important for getting a good view. Control of bleeding is achieved by increasing intra-articular pressure to above systolic blood pressure. This can be done either by elevating the head of fluid, or by the use of a pump, increasing flow to wash out the joint, or the use of 1 ml 1/100 000 adrenaline solution in 3000 ml saline for irrigation. If the exposure is not adequate, traction *must not* be increased. The procedure should be terminated and open repair undertaken.

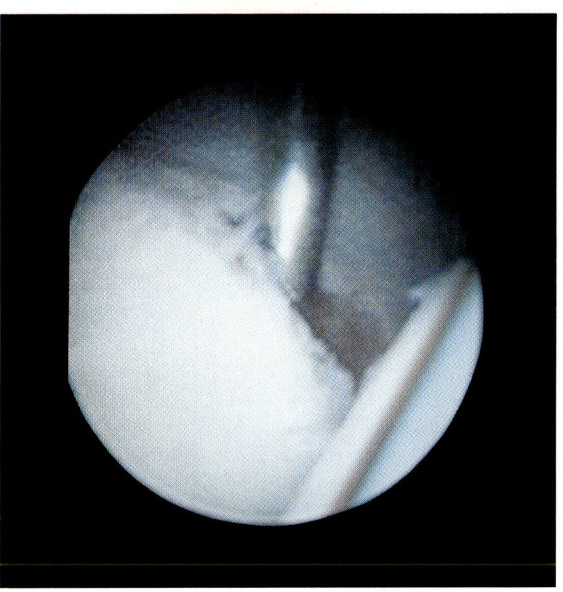

Figure 9.9
The glenoid neck is prepared using a bur.

Arthroscopic stapling method

Preparation of the bed for reattachment of the AIGHL labrum complex is vital to the success of the procedure. The Bankart lesion should be extended inferiorly so as to allow the AIGHL to be shifted upwards and medially later in the procedure. The extension of the lesion must be performed with the greatest of care, firstly in order that the AIGHL complex is not damaged further; secondly because the axillary nerve lies just inferior to the axillary fold of the IGHL. Extension of the Bankart lesion also allows better access to the front of the glenoid neck which can be prepared by using a curette, the motorized shaving system or drill holes (Figure 9.9). The idea is to create a bleeding bed, for the bed must be vascularized for healing to occur. The staple is then inserted through the anterior portal, and the superior band of the AIGHL is impaled between the tines of the staple (Figure 9.10). It is now vital that the staple, with the impaled AIGHL, is *shifted* both superiorly up the anterior glenoid rim, and then medially in front of the glenoid rim to tighten up the inferior glenohumeral ligament complex

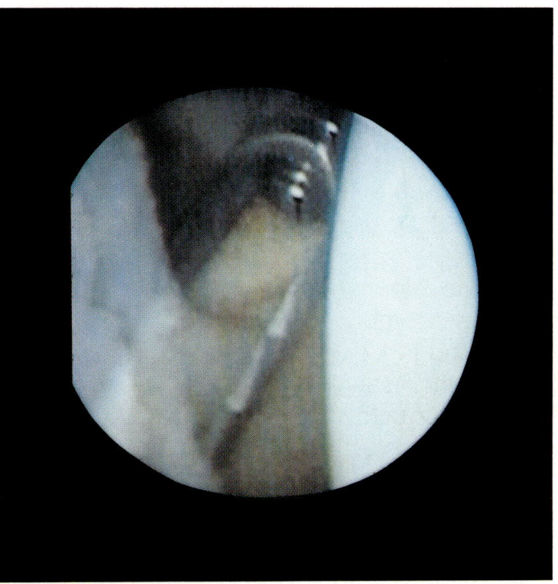

Figure 9.10
The superior band of the inferior glenohumeral ligament is impaled between the tines of the staple.

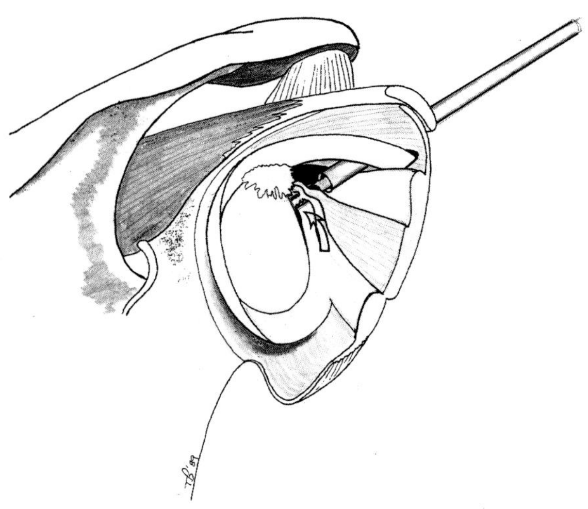

Figure 9.11
The staple is shifted upwards and medially to tighten the inferior glenohumeral ligament complex.

and place it on the previously prepared vascularized bed (Figure 9.11). The staple is then hammered home. Loose staples are usually a result of the staple not being firmly inserted at operation, and it is sometimes difficult to judge if placement is secure, as the staple lies in front of the glenoid and can only be seen correctly with the arthroscope in the anterior portal.

The staple is removable if there is a failure to secure it to the bone, misplacement, unexplained pain, repeat surgery or if in the throwing athlete. A biodegradable staple is currently being tested by Johnson.

Postoperative regime

The patient is immobilized in a sling in internal rotation for a *full* 3-week period. During weeks 4–6, pendulum exercises are encouraged. At week 7, overhead exercises are encouraged. When the patient has regained his preoperative range of motion, shoulder-strengthening exercises are started. When deltoid and cuff power have returned to preoperative levels then sports are allowed, *but no throwing is allowed for 6 months*.

Results

By the end of 1987, 195 cases had been performed and 147 had a follow-up of over 2 years. The following associated pathology was found: 13 per cent had rotator cuff tears, 90 per cent had a Hill–Sachs lesion, 4 per cent had an anterior glenoid fracture (usually small), 14 per cent had loose bodies, and 10 per cent had a posterior labral tear. All the patients had some form of Bankart lesion. In 75 per cent, this consisted of detachment of the AIGHL alone, 16 per cent had detachment of both the MGHL and AIGHL, and 9 per cent had complete absence of ligaments.

Throughout the series there was a shift from using multiple staples to using a single staple. Preparation also developed from burring to drilling the anterior glenoid neck. The following technical problems were encountered. In 9 per cent, the ligaments were inadequate, a subscapularis tenodesis was attempted but 5 out of 15 redislocated, so this procedure has been abandoned. If patients have no glenohumeral ligaments, they require open augmentation. Inadequate glenoid decortication was solved by changing the scope portal to the front or using a 90 degree arthroscope. Staple problems were encountered in the form of bending, breaking, missing the bone or loosening.

In the first 5 years, 6 months, there was no case of infection and no neurovascular injury,

Table 9.2 Results of staple anterior repair by year of surgery (Johnson[4]).

Year	*Cases*	*Lost*	*Redislocation*
1982	2	–	0
1983	16	–	3
1984	**55**	**1**	**16**
1985	36	2	3
1986	42	1	8
1987	44	–	1
Total	195	4	31 (15%)

15 staples had to be removed: 8 because of pain, 3 in athletes, 2 for loosening and 2 for poor position. The redislocation rate was 21 per cent. If the table of results is examined closely (Table 9.2), it can be seen that there was an unusually high dislocation rate in 1984. An analysis of the redislocations showed that those of 1984 were partly due to a change of postoperative policy to immobilization for only 2 weeks. This has been reinstated to 3 weeks. Two patients were AMBRI. Twenty-two patients redislocated while undertaking activities such as prizefighting, barfighting, basketball, football, baseball, waterskiing and diving.

External rotation was not limited subsequent to the procedure. Johnson, as mentioned, has made the interesting observation that external rotation is limited preoperatively, and this brings into question historical reports of normal rotation with various open procedures.

In summary the *advantages* of staple repair are: accurate diagnosis, microdebridement, lesion assessment and selective repair, which can be performed as a day-case procedure. The *disadvantages* are that it is a difficult technique, with a learning curve, and it can only be performed if the ligaments are present. The redislocation rate is 21 per cent but if short immobilization and collision sports are excluded, the redislocation rate is only 6 per cent. No extra-articular reinforcement is possible and there are staple problems. A biodegradable staple is being tested.

Arthroscopic suture repair: Morgan technique

In 1959 Viek and Ben[10] described a technique for reattaching the Bankart lesion using pullout sutures. They acknowledged Luckey with the concept. Three 0.3 cm (1/8 inch) Steinmann pins were drilled through the glenoid from the front and then out of the back of the patient, passing through infraspinatus and skin. Pullout sutures were taken through these transglenoid tunnels and tied over on the skin. The sutures were removed at 3 weeks. Morgan and Bodenstab[11] took this concept and performed the operation arthroscopically. The advantages of this technique are its simplicity, the lack of damage to the glenoid neck, and the fact that no metallic hardware is left in the joint.

Method

Set up

The patient is placed in the lateral position and the arm is suspended, using two shoulder holders, in a position of internal rotation.

Diagnostic arthroscopy

This is performed for the same reasons as in the staple repair. Bleeding is controlled by adding 1 ml 1:1000 adrenaline solution to each 3 l bag of saline.

Procedure

An anterior portal is made through which a 7 mm utility arthroscopic cannula is passed. The Bankart lesion is probed and assessed. The anterior glenoid neck is prepared exactly as for staple repair.

The arthroscopic suture is performed using a specially designed stainless steel suture pin, 2 mm in diameter and 30 cm in length. This pin has a specially sharp pointed tip which is necessary to 'pick up' the labrum. The trailing end of the suture pin has a recessed eye to carry the suture. Two passes of the suture pin are made, the lower one first. The suture pin is introduced through the 7 mm cannula into the front of the joint (Figure 9.12) and the sharp tip is used to spear the IGHL labral complex at their junction. The sharp tip of the pin can now be seen between the labrum and the prepared anterior glenoid rim (Figure 9.13) and the pin is now used to *shift* the speared soft tissue both superiorly and medially on the glenoid neck in order to tighten up the IGHL labrum complex. The pin is knocked into the prepared bone with a tap from a mallet, in a position about 3 mm medial to the glenoid neck.

It is important at this stage to angle the pin for a safe passage through the glenoid. In order to miss the suprascapular nerve on exiting the glenoid, the pin must be angled 15 degrees downward (caudad) to a line drawn perpendicular to the long axis of the glenoid. The pin must also run parallel to the articular surface of the glenoid or, at the most, 15 degrees angled in to the glenoid. Angled any less, the pin may break through into the joint and, angled any more, it might hit the suprascapular nerve (Figure 9.14). Rose has developed a guide, similar to an anterior cruciate ligament (ACL) guide, which can be used to make passage of

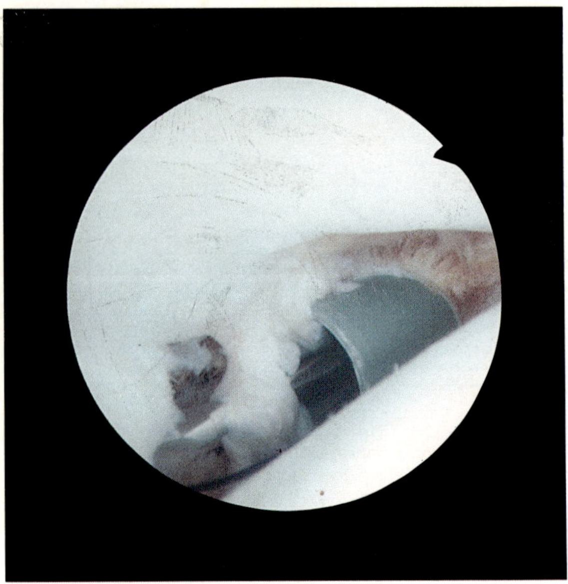

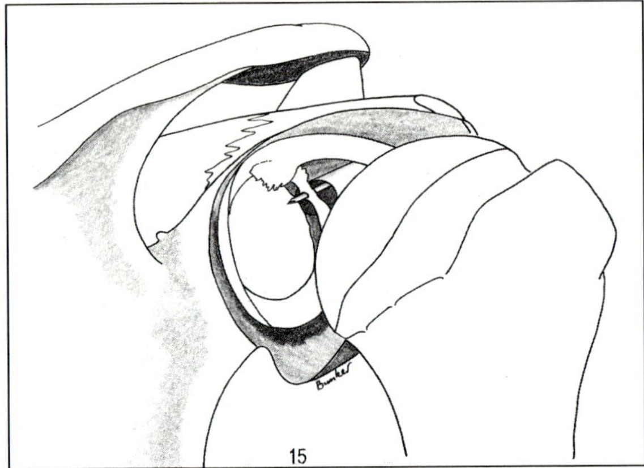

Figure 9.12

The suture pin is inserted through a 7 mm cannula into the front of the joint.

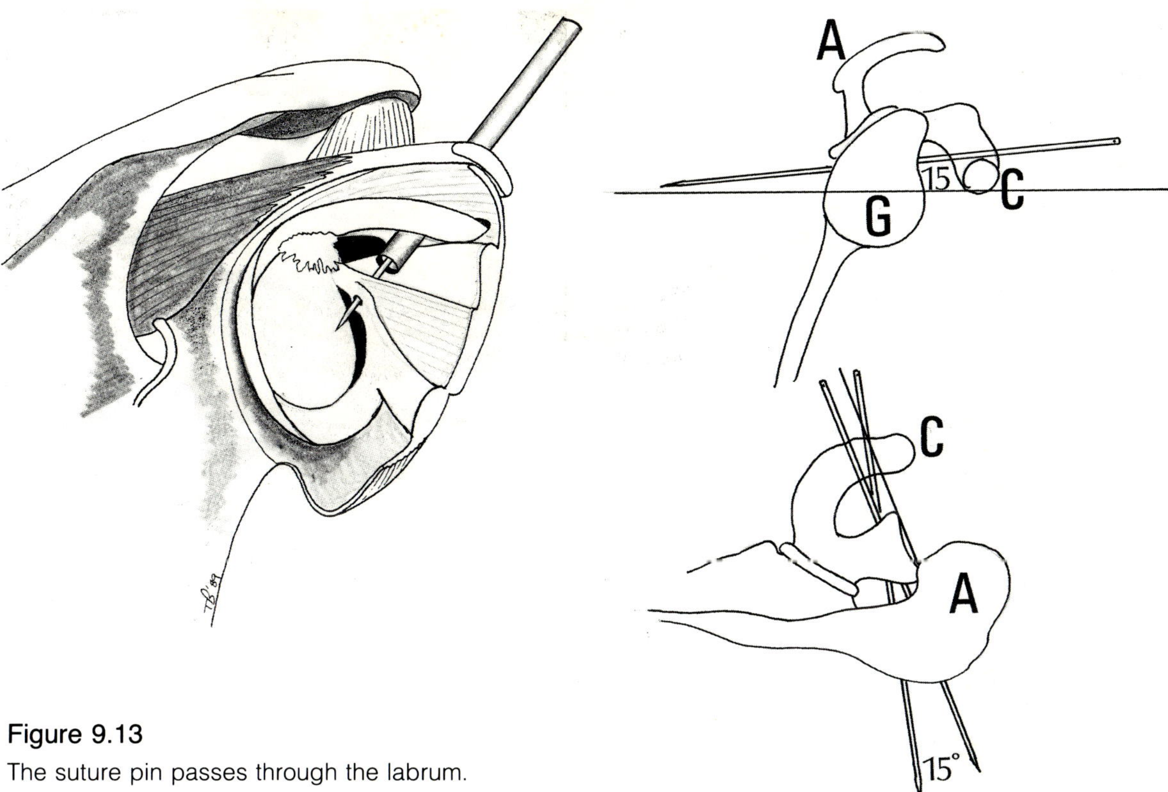

Figure 9.13

The suture pin passes through the labrum.

Figure 9.14

The suture pin should pass downward (caudad) 15 degrees, and either parallel to or 15 degrees medial to the glenoid articular surface to avoid damage to the joint surface and the suprascapular nerve.

the pins more accurate. The results are yet to be published.

The pin is then driven through the bone using a power drill and a 5 mm stab incision made over the skin at the point where the skin is tented up by the pin. The pin now passes from the front of the shoulder, through the cannula, the Bankart lesion, the glenoid and out of the back of the shoulder (Figure 9.15). A length of 1 PDS suture is passed through the eye of the suture pin and a haemostat attached to the two ends of the thread. A pair of pliers is now used to grasp the sharp end of the pin and pull it through the shoulder from the back (Figure 9.16) so that it is now replaced by a double thickness length of 1 PDS suture.

A second passage of the pin is made through the cannula piercing the Bankart lesion about

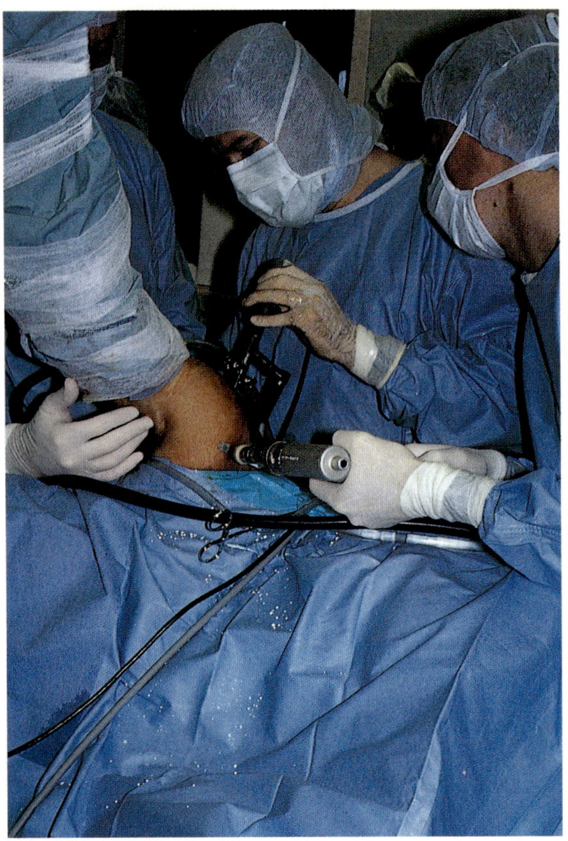

Figure 9.15
The pin is drilled through the glenoid.

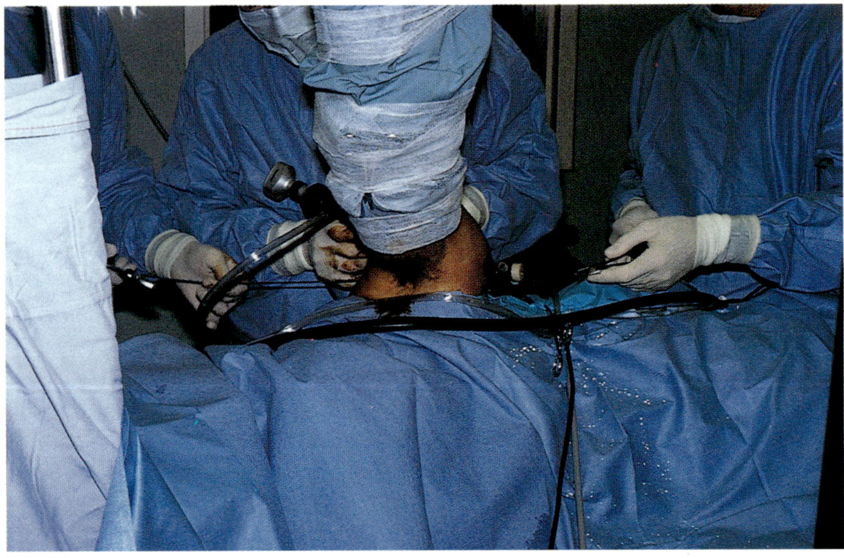

Figure 9.16
The assistant grasps the suture pin and pulls the suture out through infraspinatus and the skin.

1.5 cm above (cephalad) to the first passage. The pin is angled parallel to the first passage and drilled through the bone. It is possible to pick up the first suture on the rotating suture pin which makes a mess of tangled suture within the joint. This can be avoided either by being aware of this possibility or by using a reciprocating drill. The second pin should exit the skin about 2 cm above the first pin. Once again a length of 1 PDS is passed through the eye of the pin, and a haemostat attached to the ends. The pliers are then used to bring the second suture through the glenoid.

At this point, there are two doubled threads of 1 PDS coming out of the cannula, each with a haemostat on the end. The two doubled threads are tied together with a double square knot and the excess trimmed off (Figure 9.17). The sutures are cut from the suture pins at the back and replaced with haemostats and by pulling on these haemostats the knotted PDS suture disappears down the cannula and comes to rest on the Bankart lesion. Further tension from behind pulls the Bankart lesion down on the prepared glenoid neck where it will be held until it has healed.

The only remaining problem is what to do with the suture at the back. A small stab incision is made between the two exiting pairs of sutures and each is retrieved subcutaneously using a haemostat and brought out through the central stab. The two pairs of threads are then tied using a double square knot over the fascia of infraspinatus. A hook probe is then inserted through the cannula and the repair is tested. If all is satisfactory, the cannula and arthroscope are withdrawn and the puncture sites are closed.

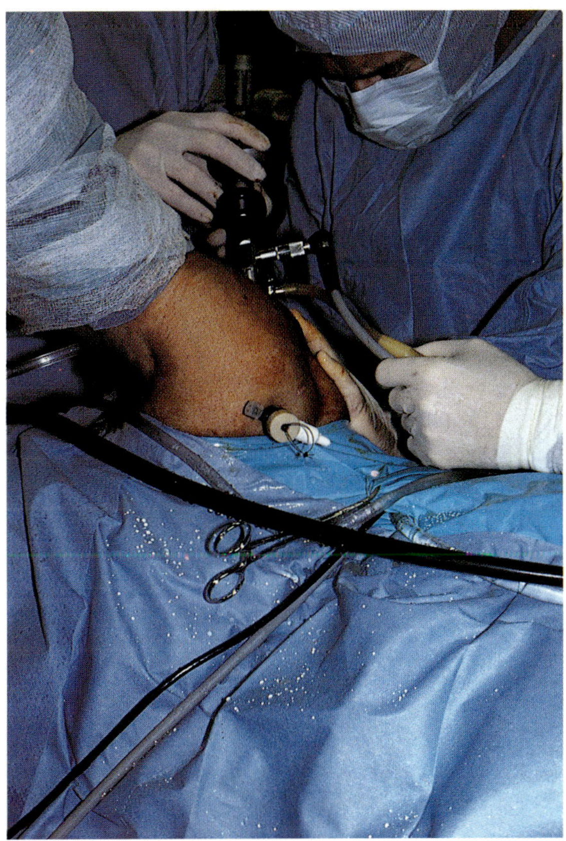

Figure 9.17

The sutures are tied together firmly and the excess cut off.

Postoperative regime

The shoulder is immobilized in internal rotation for 6 weeks. Approximately 10 days postoperatively, the skin sutures may be removed and the patient is allowed to remove the shoulder immobilizer three times daily for elbow extension exercises. The patient is allowed to shower, as long as the arm is kept in internal rotation. At 4 weeks, active assisted and Codman pendulum exercises are used under the physiotherapist's direction. At 6 weeks, TheraBand exercises are used to strengthen the rotator cuff. Vigorous exercises including contact sports and throwing are not allowed until 6 months after the repair.

Results

Morgan presented his 2–5 years results at the American Academy of Orthopaedic Surgeons' 1989 meeting.[12] Of 60 patients, 55 had a Bankart lesion, all had a positive anterior apprehension sign, and none were lax jointed or had a sulcus sign. Follow-up was graded by the Rowe assessment at an average of 37 months. There were only two failures: one redislocated playing American football, fracturing his glenoid neck at the same time, and one subluxed. One patient had a neuropraxia of the medial antebrachial cutaneous nerve, but no evidence of injury to the suprascapular nerve and no problems with the suture over infraspinatus. Of the 96 per cent graded as excellent, which is comparable to the best open series, 53 had excellent results, including 46 who achieved a full range of shoulder movement, and 7 who lacked 5 degrees of movement.

Inferior capsular shift

Caspari and Rose have each devised a method of picking up the IGHL labrum complex with a suturing device. Caspari devised a suture punch which could be used to deliver a suture through the superior band of the IGHL. The problem with the suture punch is its size, in particular withdrawing it from the front of the

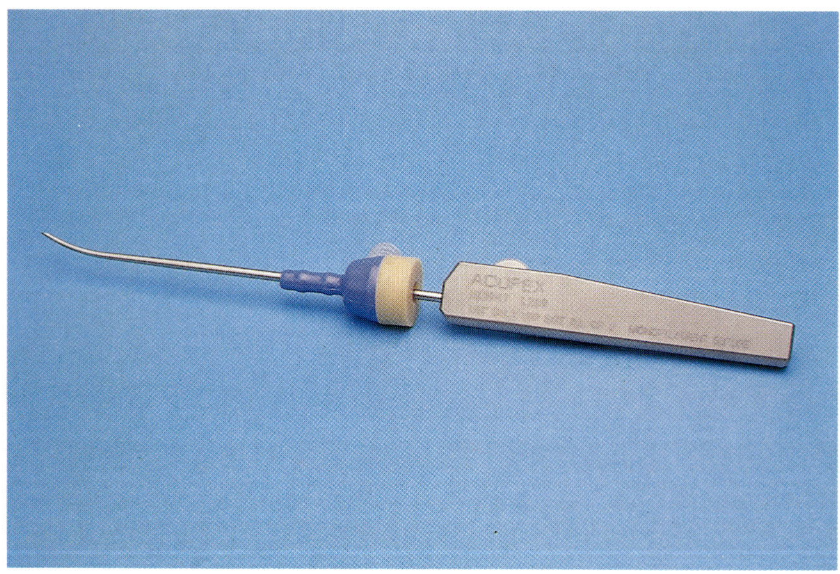

Figures 9.18 and 9.19

Rose's suture passer is used to pass a suture through the glenoid labrum.

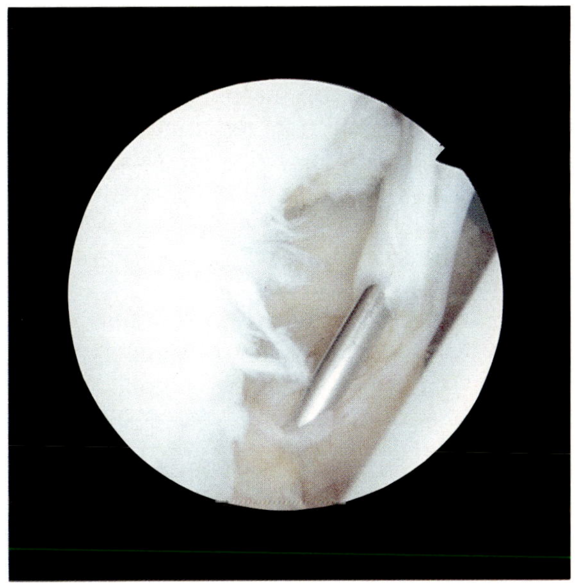

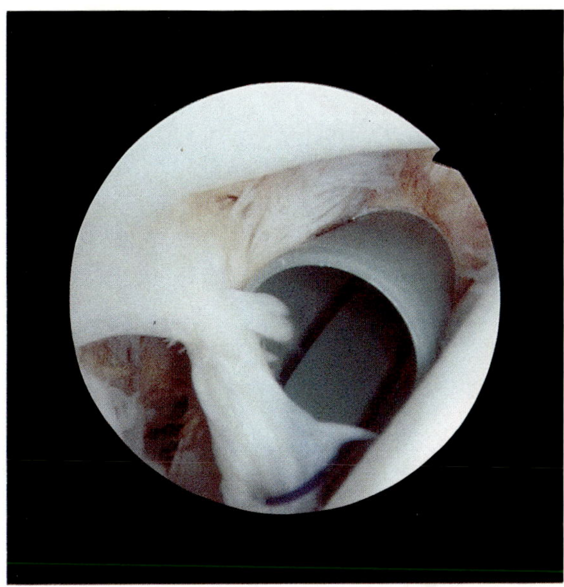

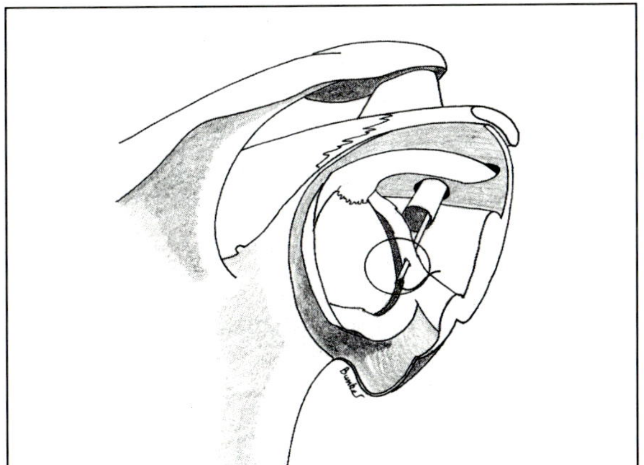

Figure 9.20

The suture placed through the labrum and exiting the cannula.

Figure 9.19

joint with its jaws open. Rose's suture passer (Figures 9.18 and 9.19) is easier to insert into the joint but needs a separate instrument to grasp the free end of the suture to withdraw it from the joint (Figure 9.20). In both techniques, the sutures, once inserted into the Bankart lesion, are passed on a suture pin through the glenoid so as to shift and tighten the IGHL labrum complex and hold it down to the prepared glenoid neck (Figure 9.21).

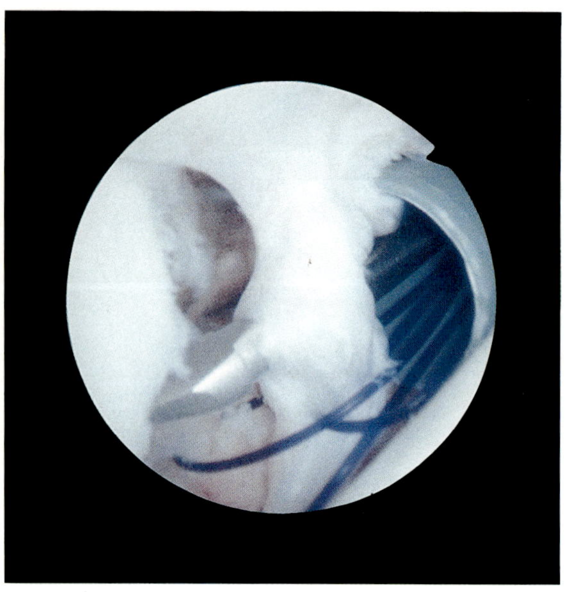

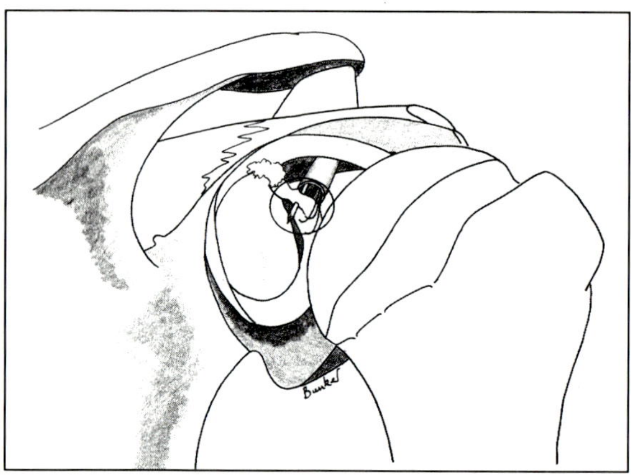

Figure 9.21

With several sutures placed, the suture pin is inserted through the prepared glenoid neck. The sutures are taken through the glenoid to be tied over the infraspinatus fascia.

Results

Caspari et al also presented their results at the American Academy of Orthopaedic Surgeons' 1989 meeting.[13] At that time they reported on 100 cases: 49 with a labral detachment had a suture repair, 51 with a midsubstance tear of the IGHL labrum complex had a semiclosed augmentation.

In the 49 suture repairs, 5–8 sutures were inserted in each patient, the maximum being 12 sutures. The patients wore an immobilizer for 3 months after surgery. The average number of preoperative dislocations was five in this group, 92 per cent had a satisfactory result, two patients had a further dislocation and two patients a further subluxation.

Of the 51 patients who had an augmentation, 80 per cent had a satisfactory result. These patients had an average of 19 preoperative episodes of dislocation, there were eight redislocations, seven in American football players, and one in a road traffic accident. This is an extremely difficult technique which is beyond the remit of this book.

References

Introduction

1. Cofield RM, Arthroscopy of the shoulder, *Mayo Clin Proc* (1983) **58**: 501–8.
2. Bunker TD, Shoulder arthroscopy, *Ann Roy Coll Surg Engl* (1989) **71**: 213–17.
3. Rowe CR, Zarins B, Recurrent transient subluxation of the shoulder, *J Bone Joint Surg* (1981) **63A**: 813–72.
4. Rockwood C, (Editorial) Shoulder arthroscopy, *J Bone Joint Surg* (1988) **70A**: 639–40.

Chapter 1

1. Klein AH, France JC, Mutschler TA, Measurement of brachial plexus strain in arthroscopy of the shoulder, *Arthroscopy* (1987) **3(1)**: 45–52.
2. Ogilvie Harris D, Arthroscopy and arthroscopic surgery of the shoulder, *Semin Orthop* (1987) **2(4)**: 246–58.
3. Matthews LS, Zarins B, Michael RH et al, Anterior portal selection for shoulder arthroscopy, *Arthroscopy* (1985) **1(1)**: 33–9.
4. Johnson LL, *Arthroscopic surgery: principles and practice* (C.V. Mosby: St Louis 1986).
5. Caspari RB, Shoulder arthroscopy: a review of the present state of the art, *Contemp Orthop* (1983) **4**: 523–30.
6. Matthews LS, Vetter WL, Helfet DL, Arthroscopic surgery of the shoulder, *Adv Orthop Surg* (1984): 203–10.
7. Bunker TD, Shoulder arthroscopy, *Ann Roy Coll Surg* (1989) **71**: 213–17.
8. Detrisac DA, Johnson LL, *Arthroscopic shoulder anatomy: pathological and surgical implications* (Slack: New Jersey 1986).
9. Neviaser TJ, Arthroscopy of the shoulder, *Orthop Clin North Am* (1987) **18(3)**: 361–72.
10. Codman EA, *The shoulder* (Todd: Boston 1934).
11. Strizak AM, Torrance LD, Jackson DW et al, Subacromial bursography, *J Bone Joint Surg* (1982) **64A**: 196–201.
12. Laumann V, Decompression of the subacromial space: an anatomical study. In Bayley I, Kessel L, eds. *Shoulder surgery* (Springer-Verlag: Berlin 1982) 14–21.
13. Matthews LS, Fadale PD, Subacromial anatomy for the arthroscopist, *Arthroscopy* (1989) **5(1)**: 36–40.
14. Matthews LS, Terry G, Vetter WL, Shoulder anatomy for the arthroscopist, *Arthroscopy* (1985) **1(2)**: 83–91.

Chapter 2

1. Hawkins RJ, Brock RM, Abrams JS et al, Acromioplasty for impingement with an intact rotator cuff, *J Bone Joint Surg* (1988) **70(A)**: 795–7.
2. Gerber G, Terrier T, Ganz R, The role of the coracoid process in the chronic impingement syndrome, *J Bone Joint Surg* (1985) **67B**: 703–8.

Chapter 3

1. Mitchell MJ, Causey G, Berthoty DP et al, Peribursal fat plane of the shoulder: anatomic study and clinical experience, *Radiology* (1988) **168**: 699–704.
2. Wallace WA, Hellier M, Improving radiographs of the injured shoulder *Radiography* (1983) **49**: 223–9.
3. Cotton RE, Rideout DF, Tears of the humeral rotator cuff: a radiological and pathological survey, *J Bone Joint Surg [Br]* (1964) **46B**: 314–28.
4. Neer CS, Anterior acromioplasty for the chronic impingement syndrome in the shoulder, *J Bone Joint Surg [Am]* (1972) **54A**: 41–50.
5. Cone RO, Resnick D, Danzig L, Shoulder impingement syndrome: radiographic evaluation, *Radiology* (1984) **150**: 29–33.
6. Hall FM, Arthrography: past, present and future, *Amer J Radiol* (1987) **149**: 561–3.
7. Lindblom K, Arthrography and roentgenography in ruptures of tendons of the shoulder joint, *Acta Radiol* (1939) **20**: 548–62.
8. Preston BJ, Jackson JP, Investigation of shoulder disability by arthrography, *Clin Radiol* (1977) **28**: 259–66.
9. Andren L, Lundberg BJ, Treatment of rigid shoulders by joint distension during arthrography, *Acta Orth Scand* (1965) **36**: 45–53.
10. Deutsch AL, Resnick D, Mink JH et al, Computed and conventional arthrotomography of the glenohumeral joint: normal anatomy and clinical experience, *Radiology* (1984) **153**: 603–9.
11. Crass JR, Craig EV, Thompson RC et al, Ultrasonography of the rotator cuff: surgical correlation, *J Clin Ultrasound* (1984) **12**: 487–92.
12. Hodler J, Fretz CJ, Terrier F et al, Rotator cuff tears: correlation of sonographic and surgical findings, *Radiology* (1988) **169**: 791–4.
13. Middleton WD, Reinus WR, Melson GL et al, Pitfalls of rotator cuff sonography, *Am J Roentgenol* (1986) **146**: 555–60.
14. Mack LA, Nyberg DA, Matsen FR III et al, Sonography of the postoperative shoulder, *Am J Roentgenol* (1988) **150**: 1089–93.
15. Kneeland JB, Carrera GF, Middleton WD et al, Rotator cuff tears: preliminary application of high-resolution MR imaging with counter rotating current loop-gap resonators, *Radiology* (1986) **160**: 695–9.
16. Huber DJ, Sauter R, Mueller E et al, MR imaging of the normal shoulder, *Radiology* (1986) **158**: 405:8.
17. Zlatkin MB, Iannotti JP, Roberts MC et al, Rotator cuff tears: diagnostic performance or MR imaging, *Radiology* (1989) **172**: 223–9.
18. Kneeland JB, Middleton WD, Carrera GF et al, MR imaging of the shoulder: diagnosis of rotator cuff tears, *Am J Roentgenol* (1987) **149**: 333–7.
19. Kieft GJ, Bloem JL, Rozing PM et al, Rotator cuff impingement syndrome: MR imaging, *Radiology* (1988) **166**: 211–14.
20. Kieft GJ, Bloem JL, Rozing PM et al, MR imaging of recurrent anterior dislocation of the shoulder, *Am J Roentgenol* (1988) **160**: 1083–7.

Chapter 4

1. Paulos LE, Chamberlain S, Murray S, Arthroscopic shoulder decompression, technique and preliminary report, *Arthroscopy* (1985) **1(2)**: 149.
2. Andrews JR, Carson WG, Ortega K, Arthroscopy of the shoulder: technique and normal anatomy, *Am J Sports Med* (1984) **12(1)**: 1–7.
3. Klein AH, France JC, Mutschler TA, Measurement of brachial plexus strain in arthroscopy of the shoulder, *Arthroscopy* (1987) **3(1)**: 45–52.

4. Caspari RB. Shoulder arthroscopy: a review of the present state of the art. *Contemp Orthop* (1982) **4**: 523–31.

5. Matthews LS, Vetter WL, Helfet DL, Arthroscopic surgery of the shoulder, *Adv Orth Surg* (1984): 203–10.

6. Matthews LS, Fadale PD. Subacromial anatomy for the arthroscopist. *Arthroscopy* (1989) **5(1)**: 36–40.

7. Gross RM, Fitzgibbons TC, Shoulder arthroscopy, a modified approach, *Arthroscopy* (1987) **1(3)**: 156–9.

8. Warren RF, Altcheck DW, Skyhar MJ et al, *Arthroscopic acromioplasty* (Presentation to American Academy of Orthopaedic Surgeons, Las Vegas 1989).

9. Skyhar MJ, Altcheck DW, Warren RF, Tips of the trade: shoulder arthroscopy in the seated position, *Orthop Rev* (1988) **17(10)**: 1033–4.

10. Rockwood CA, Shoulder arthroscopy, Editorial, *J Bone Joint Surg* (1988) **70A**: 639–40.

Chapter 5

1. Matthews LS, Terry G, Vetter WL, Shoulder anatomy for the arthroscopist, *Arthroscopy* (1985) **1(2)**: 83–91.

2. Moseley HF, Overgaard B, The anterior capsular mechanism in recurrent dislocation of the shoulder, *J Bone Joint Surg* (1962) **44B**: 913–27.

3. Turkel SJ, Panio MW, Marshall JL et al, Stabilizing mechanisms preventing anterior dislocation of the glenohumeral joint, *J Bone Joint Surg* (1981) **63A**: 1208–17.

4. O'Brien SJ, Warren RF, Anatomy and histology of the inferior glenohumeral ligament complex (Presentation to Shoulder and Elbow Surgeons' Open Meeting, Las Vegas 1989).

Chapter 6

1. Detrisac DA, Johnson LL, Arthroscopic shoulder anatomy: pathological and surgical implications (Slack: New Jersey 1986).

2. Wiley AM, *Shoulder arthroscopy*. British Orthopaedic Association Meeting, Oxford 1988.

Chapter 7

1. Bunker TD, Time for a new name for frozen shoulder, *Br Med J* (1985) **290**: 1233–4.

2. Bunker TD, Shoulder arthroscopy, *Ann Roy Coll Surg* (1989) **71(4)**: 213–18.

3. Ogilvie Harris DJ, Arthroscopy and arthroscopic surgery of the shoulder, *Semin Orthop* (1987) **2(4)**: 246–58.

4. Ha'eri GB, Maitland A, Arthroscopic findings in frozen shoulder, *J Rheumatol* (1981) **8**: 149–52.

5. Johnson LL, *Symposium: the controversy of arthroscopic versus open approaches to shoulder instability* (American Shoulder and Elbow Surgeons' Meeting, February 1988).

6. Zarins B, Prodromos CC, Shoulder injuries in sports. In Carter Rowe ed. *The Shoulder* (Churchill Livingstone: New York 1988) 411–33.

7. Andrews JR, Carson WG, Mcleod WD, Glenoid labrum tears related to the long head of the biceps, *Am J Sports Med* (1985) **13(5)**: 337–41.

Chapter 8

1. Gerber G, Terrier T, Ganz R, The role of the coracoid process in the chronic impingement syndrome, *J Bone Joint Surg* (1985) **67(B)**: 703–8.

2. Matthews LS, Fadale PD, Subacromial anatomy for the arthroscopist, *Arthroscopy* (1989) **5(1)**: 36–40.

3. Sigholm G, Styf J, Korner L. et al, Pressure recording in the subacromial bursa, *J Orthop Res* (1988) **6(1)**: 123–8.

4. Hawkins RJ, Abrams JS, Impingement syndrome in the absence of rotator cuff tear, *Orthop Clin North Am* (1987) **18**: 373–82.

5. Neer CS, Anterior acromioplasty for the chronic impingement syndrome in the shoulder, *J Bone Joint Surg* (1972) **54(A)**: 41–50.

6. Chard MD, Sattelle LM, Hazleman BL, The long-term outcome of rotator cuff tendinitis – a review study, *Br J Rheumatol* (1988) **27(5)**: 385–9.
7. Ellman H, Kay SP, Arthroscopic subacromial decompression: 2 to 5 year results (Presentation, American Shoulder and Elbow Surgeons, Open Meeting, February 1989).
8. Alcheck DW, Schwartz E, Warren RF et al, Arthroscopic acromioplasty, *Arthroscopy* (1988) **4(2)**: 145.
9. Ellman H, Arthroscopic subacromial decompression: analysis of 1 to 3 year results, *Arthroscopy* (1987) **3(3)**: 173–81.
10. Gartsman GM, Blair ME, Noble PC et al, Arthroscopic subacromial decompression: an anatomical study, *Am J Sports Med* (1988) **16(1)**: 48–50.
11. Warren RF, Altcheck DW, Skyhar MJ et al, Arthroscopic acromioplasty (Presentation to American Academy Orthopaedic Surgeons' Meeting, Las Vegas 1989).

Chapter 9

1. Matsen FA, in Matsen FA and Rockwood CA, eds. *The Shoulder* (WB Saunders: Philadelphia, 1990), p. 151.
2. Rowe CR, Patel D, Southmayd WW, The Bankart procedure: a long-term end result study, *J Bone Joint Surg* (1978) **60A**: 1–16.
3. Hovelius L, Eriksson G, Fredin F et al, Recurrences after initial dislocation of the shoulder, *J Bone Joint Surg* (1983) **65A**: 343–9.
4. Johnson LL, Symposium: the controversy of arthroscopic vs open approaches to shoulder instability. (Presentation to American Shoulder and Elbow Surgeons, Meeting, February 1988).
5. Turkel SJ, Panio MW, Marshall JL et al, Stabilizing mechanisms preventing anterior dislocation of the glenohumeral joint, *J Bone Joint Surg* (1981) **63(A)**: 1208–17.
6. O'Brien SJ, Neves M, Rozbruch R et al, Anatomy and histology of the inferior glenohumeral ligament complex (Presentation to American Shoulder and Elbow Surgeons' Open Meeting, Las Vegas 1989).
7. Oveison J, Nielson S, Anterior and posterior shoulder instability. *Acta Orthop Scand* (1986) **57**: 324–47.
8. Du Toit GT, Roux D, Recurrent dislocation of the shoulder: a 24 year study of the Johannesburg stapling operation. *J Bone Joint Surg* (1956) **38A**: 1–12.
9. Boyd HB, Hunt HL, Recurrent dislocation of the shoulder, *J Bone Joint Surg* **47A**: 1514–20.
10. Viek P, Ben BT, The Bankart shoulder reconstruction: the use of pull out wires and other details, *J Bone Joint Surg* (1959) **41A**: 236–42.
11. Morgan CD, Bodenstab AB, Arthroscopic suture repair: technique and early results, *Arthroscopy* (1987) **3(2)**: 111–22.
12. Morgan CD, Arthroscopic Bankart suture repair, 2 to 5 year results (Presentation to American Shoulder and Elbow Surgeons' Open Meeting, Las Vegas 1989).
13. Caspari RB, Savoie FH, Meyers JF, Arthroscopic management of the unstable shoulder (Presentation to American Academy Orthopaedic Surgeons, Las Vegas 1989).

Further reading

Andrews J, Broussard T, Carson W, Arthroscopy of the shoulder in the management of partial tears of the rotator cuff, *Arthroscopy* (1985) **1((2)**:117–22.

Bjorkenheim JM, Paavolainen P, Ahovue J et al, Surgical repair of the rotator cuff and surrounding tissues: factors influencing the results, *Clin Orthop* (1988) Nov(**236**):148–53.

Bryan WJ, Schauder K, Tullos HS, The axillary nerve and its relationship to common sports medicine shoulder procedures, *Am J Sports Med* (1986) **14(2)**:113–6.

Burman MS, Arthroscopy or direct visualization of joints, *J Bone Joint Surg* (1931) **13**:669–95.

Cofield RH, Irving JF, Evaluation and classification of shoulder instability, with special reference to examination under anaesthesia, *Clin Orthop* (1987) Oct(**223**):32–43.

Dolk T, Gremark O, Arthroscopy and stability testing of the shoulder joint, *Arthroscopy* (1986) **2(1)**:35–40.

Ellman H, Shoulder arthroscopy: current indications and techniques, *Orthopedics* (1988) **11(1)**:45–51.

Esch JC, Ozerkis LR, Helgager JA et al, Arthroscopic subacromial decompression, *Arthroscopy* (1988) **4(2)**:138.

Gregg JR, Torg E, Upper extremity injuries in adolescent tennis players, *Clin Sports Med* (1988) **7(2)**:371–85.

Howell SM, Galinet BJ, Renz AJ et al, Normal and abnormal mechanics of the glenohumeral joint in the horizontal plane, *J Bone Joint Surg* (1988) **70(2)A**:227–32.

Kujat R, The microangiographic pattern of the glenoid labrum of the dog, *Arch Orthop Trauma Surg* (1986) **105(5)**:310–2.

Lilleby H, Shoulder arthroscopy, *Acta Orthop Scand* (1984) **55(5)**:561–6.

Matthews LS, Oweida SJ, Glenohumeral instability in athletes: spectrum, diagnosis and treatment, *Adv Orthop Surg* (1985) 236–49.

Matthews LS, Vetter WL, Oweida SJ et al, Arthroscopic staple capsulloraphy for recurrent anterior instability, *Arthroscopy* (1988) **4(2)**:106–11.

McMaster WC, Anterior glenoid labrum damage: a painful lesion in swimmers, *Am J Sports Med* (1986) **14(5)**:383–7.

McGlynn FJ, Caspari RB, Arthroscopic findings in the subluxating shoulder, *Clin Orthop* (1984) **183**:173–8.

Oretorp N, Bassi PB, Arthroscopy of the shoulder joint (technique), *Ital J Orthop Traumatol* (1983) **9(2)**:251–8.

Ozaki J, Glenohumeral movements of the involuntary inferior and multidirectional instability, *Clin Orthop* (1989) **238**:107–11.

Parisien JS, Shoulder arthroscopy: technique and indications, *Bull Hosp Jt Dis Orthop Inst* (1983) **43(1)**:56–69.

Thorling J, Bjernald H, Hallin G et al, Acromioplasty for impingement syndrome, *Acta Orthop Scanda* (1985) **56(2)**:147–8.

Tibone JE, Jobe FW, Kerlan RK et al, Shoulder impingement syndrome in athletes treated by an anterior acromioplasty, *Clin Orthop* (1985) Sep(**198**):134–40.

Tibone JE, Prietto C, Jobe FW, Staple capsulorraphy for recurrent posterior dislocation, *Am J Sports Med* (1981) **9**:135–9.

Uhthoff HK, Hammond DI, Sarker K et al, The role of the coracoacromial ligament in the impingement syndrome: a clinical, radiological and histological study, *Int Orthop* (1988) **12(2)**:97–104.

Waldron VD, Technique of shoulder arthroscopy, *Orthop Rev* (1988) **17(6)**:652–5.

Wiley AM, Older MWJ, Shoulder arthroscopy, *Am J Sports Med* (1980) **8(1)**:31–8.

Wiley AM, Arthroscopy for shoulder instability and a technique for arthroscopic repair, *Arthroscopy* (1988) **4(1)**:25–30.

Wiley AM, Arthroscopic shoulder surgery, *Surg Endosc* (1987) **1(1)**:65–9.

Wolf W, Arthroscopic anterior staple capsulorraphy, *Arthroscopy* (1988) **4(2)**:142.

Zuckerman JD, Matsen FA, Complications about the glenohumeral joint related to the use of screws and staples, *J Bone Joint Surg* (1984) **66A**:175–81.

Index

Acromioclavicular pain, 25
  effect of adduction test, 36
  painful arc, 28
Acromion, angle, anatomy, 9
Adduction test, 36
  effect on acromioclavicular joint, 36
Anaesthesia, examination under, 2
Anaesthesia for shoulder arthroscopy, 58–59
  general, 59
  local, 58
  scalene block, 58
Anterior apprehension test, 36
Anterior drawer test, 36
Anterior reconstruction of traumatic instabilities, five-year results, 6
Arm and shoulder positions during arthroscopy, 56–58
Arthritis, arthroscopic examination, 109, 117, 118
Arthrobot, 56
Arthrodesis, 129
Arthrography, shoulder, 44–46
  computerized tomography, 46–47
  digital subtraction, 47
Arthroscope technique
  bursal endoscopy, 72–73
  cannulation, 70
  inside-out technique, 70–72
  introducing needle, 64–69
  outside-in technique, 70
Arthroscopic examination, abnormal findings, 99–121
  arthritis, 109, 117, 118
  biceps, long head, 99
    tendon, 100, 101
  fractures, 118–119, 120
  glenohumeral ligament, 109, 111
  glenoid labrum, 99, 106–109
  Hill–Sachs lesions, 109, 112–116
  inferior glenohumeral ligament complex, 99, 106–108
  inferior glenohumeral recess, 109
  joint replacement, 119–121
  labral tears, 109
  posterior labrum, 109
  rotator cuff, 99, 102
  shoulder sepsis, 121
  synovium, 109
Arthroscopic examination, normal findings, 75–97
  bursoscopy, 94–97
  glenohumeral ligaments, 85–94
  hook probe, 89
  long head of biceps, 76–82
  normal track, 75
  rotator cuff, 82
  subscapularis tendon, 83–85
Arthroscopic staple repair, 145–149
  associated lesions, 146
  diagnostic arthroscopy, 146
Arthroscopic staple repair (*cont.*)
  examination under anaesthesia, 146
  exposure, 147
  postoperative regime, 148
  results, 148–149
  stapling method, 147
Arthroscopic subacromial decompression, 131–140
  anatomy, subacromial space, 131–134
  diagnosis, 134–135
    algorithm, 135
  Ellman method, 136–139
  impingement, 131–134
  indications for surgery, 134–135
  learning curve, 6
  open or closed surgery, 134
  postoperative management, 139–140
  results, 140
Arthroscopic surgery, 6–7, 123–130
  fifth generation surgery, 6, 129–130
    arthrodesis, 129
    rotator cuff repair, 130
  first generation, 6, 123–128
    diagnostic arthroscopy, 123
    labral tears, excision, 128
    loose bodies, removal, 125–127
    targeted biopsy, 123–125
  five subdivisions, 6

Arthroscopic surgery (*cont.*)
  fourth generation surgery, 6, 123
  future trends, 7
  general features, 6–7
  second generation, 6, 128–129
    arthroscopic subacromial decompression, 128, 131–140, *see also* Arthroscopic subacromial decompression
    coracoacromial ligament division, 129
    cuff tears, 129
    osteoarthritis, 129
    shoulder debridement, 129
    synovectomy, 129
  third generation surgery, 6, 123
  training, 6, 7, 51
Arthroscopic suture repair, 149–154
  Morgan technique, 149–154
    postoperative regime, 153–155
    procedure, 150–153
    results, 154
Arthroscopy
  diagnostic, 123
  disorders most helped, 1–5
  indications, 1–5
Axillary artery, anatomy, 16–20
Axillary nerve, anatomy, 9–12

Bankart lesion, 1–2
  differentiation from labral tear, 128
  glenoid/labrum separation, 106, 107
  repair, success rate, 6
  surgery, 142, 143, 145
Biceps
  anatomy, 15
  long head, arthroscopic examination, 76–82
  synovial adhesion, 76
  synovial infold, 76
  tendon, abnormal findings, 100, 101
Biopsy, targeted, in arthroscopic surgery, 123–125
Bursal endoscopy, 72–73
Bursoscopy, 94–97

Calcification, soft tissue, X-ray, 42
Capsule, shoulder *see* Shoulder capsule
Caspari punch, 54
Circumflex capsular artery, anatomy, 13
Clicking during examination, 32
Clinical procedure, 51–73
  equipment, 52–54, *see also* Equipment
  normal arthroscopic examination, 75–97
  preoperative, 58–70, *see also* Preoperative procedures
  theatre organization, 51–52
Computerized tomography arthography, 46–47
Coracoacromial ligament division, 129, 138

Deltoid muscle, anatomy, 9
Diagnosis, 1–5
Digital subtraction arthrography, 47
Dislocation, traumatic, shoulder, 141–156
  arthroscopic management, 141–156
    arthroscopic staple repair, 1475–149
    arthroscopic suture repair, 149–154
    atraumatic multidirectional bilateral rehabilitation shift, 141
    inferior capsular shift, 154–156
    recurrence following dislocation, 141
    recurrent anterior dislocation, 142–145
    traumatic unidirectional Bankart surgery, 141, 143
Electrosurgical apparatus, subacromial decompression, 53–54
Ellman method, subacromial decompression, 136–139
Endoscopy, bursal, 72–73
Equipment, 52–58
  for arthroscopic photography, 54
  for arthroscopic surgery of shoulder, 52–54
  for diagnostic shoulder arthroscopy, 52
  shoulder holders, 56–58
Examination, shoulder girdle, 29–36
  active movements, 33–34
  adduction test, 36
  arthroscopic *see* Arthroscopic examination
  'feel', 33
  impingement tests, 36
  instability tests, 36–39
  'look', 32
  'move', 33–36
  passive movements, 34
  rotator cuff strength, 34–36
  self-assessment sheet, 30–31
  under anaesthetic, 2
Extrascapular anatomy, 9–24

Failed previous shoulder surgery, indication for arthroscopy, 6
Fractures, arthroscopic examination, 118–119, 120
Frozen shoulder, 124–125

Glenohumeral ligaments
  abnormal findings, 109, 111
  normal, 85–94
    rotation of arthroscope, 89
    superior/middle/inferior, anatomy, 85–89
  in recurrent anterior dislocation, 142
  stapling, 147
Glenohumeral pain, 25
Glenohumeral recess, inferior, 109

Glenoid labrum, abnormal arthroscopic findings, 99, 106–108, 109

Hairy degeneration, rotator cuff, 2
Hatchet lesion, X-ray, 43
Hill–Sachs lesions, 2, 109, 112–116, 142, 143
Humerus, anatomy, 14

Imaging the shoulder, 41–50
  arthrography, 44–46
  CT arthrography, 46–47
  digital subtraction arthrography, 47
  magnetic resonance imaging, 49–50
  plain radiography, 41–44
  subacromial bursography, 47
  techniques, 41
  ultrasound, 47–49
Impingement
  injection test, 34, 36
  lesion, 2
  syndrome, 131–134
    subacromial space, anatomy, 131–132
Indications, 1–5
Inferior capsular shift, 154–155
  results, 155
  Rose's suture passer, 154, 155
  1GHL labrum complex, 154
Inferior glenohumeral ligament complex, abnormal arthroscopic findings, 99, 106–108
Inferior glenohumeral recess, abnormal findings, 109
Infraspinatus muscle, arthroscopic track, 12
  insertions, 2
  reflected, 13
  test, 35
Inside-out technique, 70
Instability tests, 36–39
Instrument Makar staples, 54

Joint replacement, arthroscopic examination, 119–121

Labral tears, 109, 110
  differentiation from Bankart lesions, 128
  excision, 128
  trimming, success rate, 6
Labrum, posterior, 109
Local anaesthesia for shoulder arthroscopy, 58
Loose bodies, arthroscopic examination, 112–116
  removal, 125–127
    success rate, 6

Magnetic resonance imaging, shoulder, 49–50
Magnusson Stack repair, success rate, 6
Metal implants, around shoulder joints, contraindications, 6–7
Morgan method, arthroscopic suture repair, 149–154
Movements, shoulder examination
  active, 33–34
  passive, 34
Muscle wasting, 32

Needle, introducing from posterior portal, 64–69
  cannulation, 69
Nerve palsies after arthroscopy, 56
Neurological assessment, 38
Nottingham axial view, shoulder X-ray, 44

Osteoarthritis, debridement, 129
Outside-in technique, 70

Pain, shoulder, assessment, 25–29
  acromioclavicular, 25
    painful arc, 28
  atypical, 2–4
  composite painful arc, 28
  definition of 'true' pain, 25
  glenohumeral, 25
  movement which exacerbates, 27–29

Pain, shoulder, assessment (*cont.*)
  referred, 25
  severity and function, 29
  specific questions to patient, 29
  specific tests, 34–39
  subacromial, 25
    painful arc, 28
  types, 25
  when it started and how, 25–27
Palpation, shoulder, 32
Paraesthesias, transient, after arthroscopy, 56
Photography, arthroscopic, 54
Portal
  anterior, anatomical landmarks, 16–20
    arthroscopic track, 16
  posterior, anatomical landmarks, 9–15
    arthroscopic directions, 9–11
    arthroscopic track, 11–15
    introducing needle, 64–69
  superior, anatomical landmarks, 20–21
    arthroscopic track, 20–21
    irrigation, 70–71
Posterior stress test, 38
Preoperative procedures, 58–70
  anaesthesia, 58–59
  draping the patient, 60–64
  inside-out technique, 70–72
  introducing the needle, 64–69
  outside-in technique, 70
  positioning, 59–60
  surgical landmarks, 63

Quadrilateral space, anatomy, 11

Radiography, shoulder, 41–44
Recurrent shoulder discomfort following trauma, 1
Rose's suture passer, 154, 155
Rotator cuff
  arthroscopic examination
    abnormal, 99–102

Rotator cuff (*cont.*)
normal, 82
tears, 103, 104, 105
repairs, 4, 6, 129–130
strength, 34–36
impingement injection test, 34
infraspinatus test, 35
subscapularis test, 35
supraspinatus test, 34
tears, 2
subacromial crepitus, 32
X-ray, 43

Scalene block for shoulder arthroscopy, 58
Scapular anastomosis, anatomy, 13
Self-assessment sheet, shoulder, 30–31
Sepsis, shoulder, arthroscopic examination, 121
Shift and load test, 36
Shoulder
and arm positions after arthroscopy, 56
assessment, 25–39
examination, 29–36, *see also* Examination
neurological assessment, 38
pain, 25–29, *see also* Pain, shoulder
Shoulder (*cont.*)
self-assessment sheet, 30–31
specific tests, 34–39
capsule, anatomy, 15
relation to axillary nerve, 11
debridement, arthroscopic surgery, 131
girdle, examination, 29–36
positions during arthroscopy, 56–58
Snapping during examination, 32
Subacromial
bursa, anatomy, 22–23
bursography, 47
crepitus, 32
decompression, 53–54
'beach-chair' position, 60
electronic apparatus, 54
impingement, chronic, 1
injection test, 34
pain, 25
painful arc, 28
space, anatomical landmarks, 21–23
anatomy, 131–134
decompression, 131–140
Subscapularis
muscle, in recurrent anterior dislocation, 142
tendon, arthroscopic examination, 83–85
Subscapularis (*cont.*)
test, 35–36
Sulcus sign, 38
Superior synovial syndrome, 124
Suprascapular artery, anatomy, 12, 13
Suprascapular nerve, anatomy, 12, 13
Supraspinatus, insertions, 2–4
Supraspinatus test, 34
Synovectomy, arthroscopic surgery, 129
Synovial adhesion, 76
Synovitis, arthroscopic examination, 109

Television system, theatre, 52–54
Tendinitis, long head of biceps, 3
Teres minor, reflected, 13
Theatre organization, 51–52, *see also* Equipment
Training for arthroscopy, 6, 7, 51

Ultrasound, shoulder, 47–49

Wissinger rod, 70

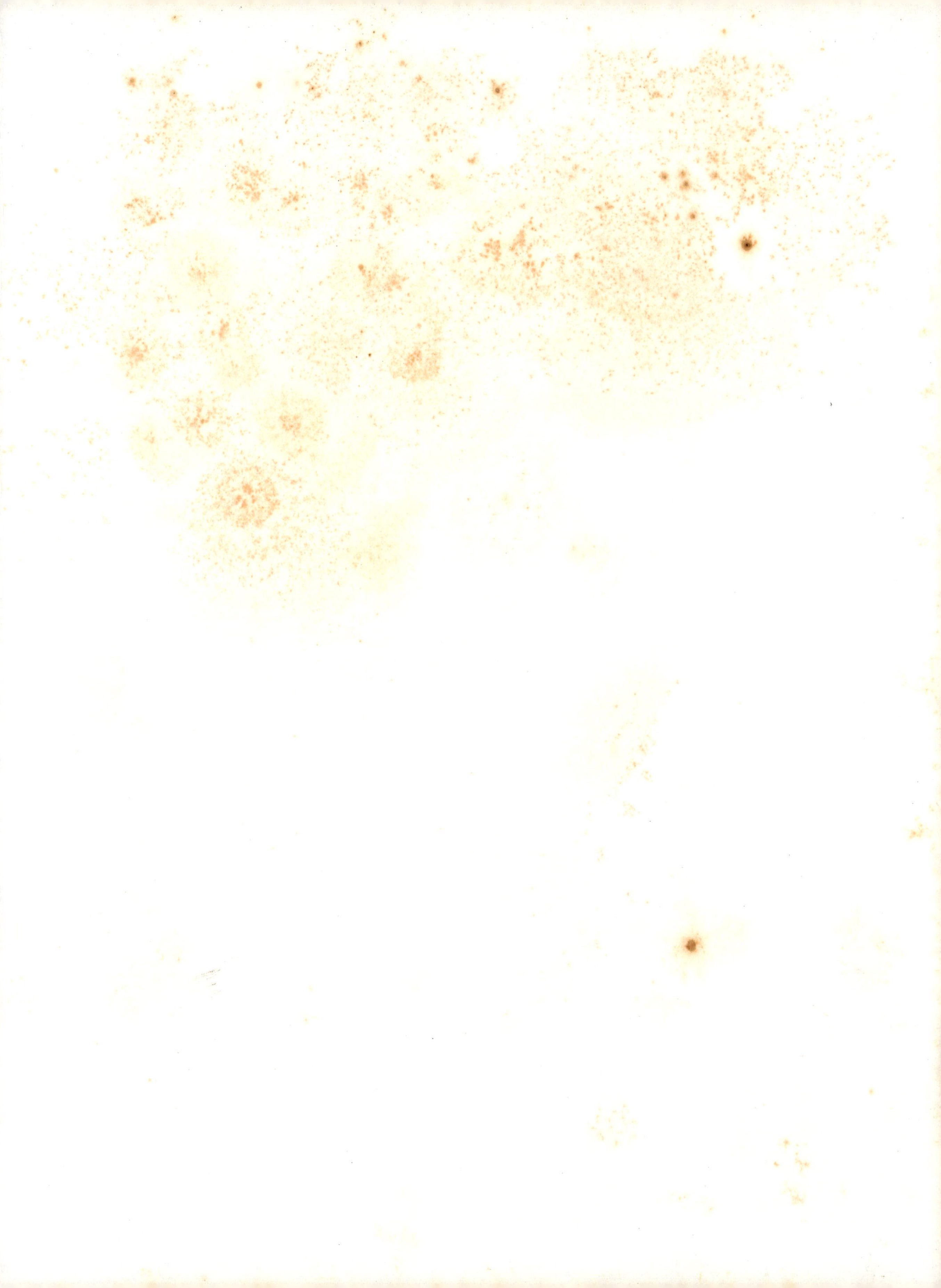